Theorising Social Exclusion

Theorising Social Exclusion first reviews and reflects upon existing thinking, literature and research into social exclusion and social connectedness, outlining an integrated theory of social exclusion across dimensions of social action and along pathways of social processes. A series of commissioned chapters then develop and illustrate the theory by addressing the machinery of social exclusion and connectedness, the pathways towards exclusion and, finally, experiences of exclusion and connection.

This innovative book takes a truly multidisciplinary approach and focuses on the often-neglected cultural and social aspects of exclusion. It will be of interest to academics and practitioners in fields of public health, health promotion, social work, community development, occupational therapy, policy, sociology, politics and environment.

The editors are all based in the School of Health and Social Development, Deakin University, where:

Ann Taket holds a Chair in Health and Social Exclusion and is Director of the Centre for Health through Action on Social Exclusion.

Beth R. Crisp is Associate Professor of Social Work.

Annemarie Nevill is Associate Lecturer in Public Health and Health Promotion.

Greer Lamaro is Associate Lecturer in Public Health and Health Promotion.

Melissa Graham is Senior Lecturer in Health Research and Epidemiology.

Sarah Barter-Godfrey is a Researcher in Public Health.

Theorising Social Exclusion

Ann Taket, Beth R. Crisp,
Annemarie Nevill, Greer Lamaro,
Melissa Graham and Sarah Barter-Godfrey

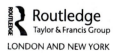

Routledge
Taylor & Francis Group

LONDON AND NEW YORK

First published 2009
by Routledge
2 Park Square, Milton Park, Abingdon, Oxon, OX14 4RN

Simultaneously published in the USA and Canada
by Routledge
270 Madison Ave, New York NY 10016

Routledge is an imprint of the Taylor & Francis Group, an informa business

Transferred to Digital Printing 2010

Typeset in Times New Roman by
Taylor & Francis Books

British Library Cataloguing in Publication Data
A catalogue record for this book is available from the British Library

Library of Congress Cataloging in Publication Data
Theorising social exclusion / Ann Taket ... [et al.].
    p. cm.
Includes bibliographical references and index.
1. Social isolation. I. Taket, A. R. (Ann R.)
HM1131.T35 2009
302.5′45–dc22
                                                          2009001282

ISBN10: 0-415-47584-8 (hbk)
ISBN10: 0-415-47585-6 (pbk)
ISBN10: 0-203-87464-1 (ebk)

ISBN13: 978-0-415-47584-6 (hbk)
ISBN13: 978-0-415-47585-3 (pbk)
ISBN13: 978-0-203-87464-6 (ebk)

Contents

List of Authors

Sarah Barter-Godfrey is a Research Fellow in the School of Health and Social Development, Deakin University, Australia.

Gemma E. Carey is currently in the School of Social and Political Sciences at the University of Melbourne, Australia.

Nicole Carvill was a PhD student in the School of Health and Social Development, Deakin University, Australia.

Kay Cook is a Senior Research Fellow in the School of Psychology, Deakin University, Australia.

Beth R. Crisp is Associate Professor in Social Work in the School of Health and Social Development, Deakin University, Australia.

Nena Foster is a Lecturer in Public Health and Health Promotion in the School of Health and Social Development, Deakin University, Australia.

Melissa Graham is a Senior Lecturer in Public Health and Health Promotion in the School of Health and Social Development, Deakin University, Australia.

Claire Henderson-Wilson is a lecturer in Public Health and Health Promotion in the School of Health and Social Development, Deakin University, Australia.

Claire Jennings is Program Manager Reading Discovery at Community Connections Victoria Ltd.

Greer Lamaro is an Associate Lecturer in Public Health and Health Promotion in the School of Health and Social Development, Deakin University, Australia.

Selma Macfarlane is a Lecturer in Social Work in the School of Health and Social Development, Deakin University, Australia.

Jane Maidment is a Senior Lecturer in Social Work in the School of Health and Social Development, Deakin University, Australia.

Erik Martin was an honours student in the School of Health and Social Development, Deakin University, Australia.

Annemarie Nevill is an Associate Lecturer in Public Health and Health Promotion in the School of Health and Social Development, Deakin University, Australia.

Janet Owens is a Senior Lecturer in Disability Studies in the School of Health and Social Development, Deakin University, Australia.

Maria Pallotta-Chiarolli is a Senior Lecturer in Social Diversity and Health in the School of Health and Social Development, Deakin University, Australia.

Bob Pease is Professor of Social Work in the School of Health and Social Development, Deakin University, Australia.

Andre M.N. Renzaho is a Senior Research Fellow in the School of Psychology, Deakin University, Australia.

Sally Savage is a Senior Research Fellow in the School of Nursing, Deakin University, Australia.

Julia Shelley is a Senior Lecturer in Social Epidemiology and Health Inequalities in the School of Health and Social Development, Deakin University, Australia.

Karen Stagnitti is an Associate Professor in Occupational Therapy in the School of Health and Social Development, Deakin University, Australia.

Ann Taket is Professor of Health and Social Exclusion in the School of Health and Social Development, Deakin University, Australia.

List of Illustrations

Figures

Tables

Boxes

PART 1

Introducing theories of social exclusion and social connectedness

1.1 Introduction

Overview

This research-based book is aimed at a wide range of different readerships globally. The book addresses issues of concern for those engaged in debates about the provision of health and social welfare services, the case for collective responsibilities, and the public service ethos more generally. Our focus is particularly upon the role of social and cultural factors in the creation and re-creation of categories of exclusion and inclusion; this finds relevance in a wide range of fields (health sciences, public health, health promotion, occupational therapy, disability studies, social work and social policy). The exploration of implications for policy and practice will make the book of relevance to a practitioner audience as well to academics.

It would not be an exaggeration to say that there are a plethora of books on social exclusion. Why another? The outline above indicates the particular approach that we wish to take, which we believe is not covered in any depth in any of the competing titles. Most of the existing titles are very strongly focused in terms of discipline and/or geography, for example (we could extend this list to several times its current length): Pierson (2001), Collins (2003), Weiss (2003), MacDonald (2004), Levitas (2005), Williams *et al.* (2005), Feldman (2006), Harness Goodwin (2006), Ryan (2007). Others, while being more multidisciplinary in approach, focus on the economistic aspects of social exclusion and do not fully address the important role of cultural and social factors in creating and re-creating categories of inclusion and exclusion, for example: Byrne (2005) and Hills *et al.* (2002). Few seek to address both issues of theory and professional practice.

The concept of social exclusion attempts to help us make sense out of the lived experience arising from multiple deprivations and inequities experienced by people and localities, across the social fabric, and the mutually reinforcing effects of reduced participation, consumption, mobility, access, integration, influence and recognition. The language of social exclusion recognises marginalising, silencing, rejecting, isolating, segregating and disenfranchising as the machinery of exclusion, its processes of operation. By way of contrast, the language of social connectedness recognises acceptance, opportunity, equity, justice, citizenship, expression and validation as the machinery of connectedness. As we will argue later, we see connectedness as the preferred conceptualisation of the opposite of exclusion, finding the concepts of inclusion and participation problematic both theoretically and in terms of policy formulation and implementation.

This book works from a multidisciplinary and intersectoral approach across health, welfare and education, linking practice and research to our growing understanding of the processes and principles that foster exclusion. We develop existing theories of exclusion and connectedness through reflection, analysis and commentary, across international perspectives and experiences recognising both global and local issues. Our focus on the role of cultural and social factors in theorising social exclusion implies a particular focus on the psychological, individual and symbolic elements of exclusion as experienced by different groups.

In this first part of the book, we review and reflect on existing thinking, literature and research into social exclusion and social connectedness. Theories of exclusion are developed concentrically across areas of action and experience, moving from the person as an excluded/connected agent, through structural, shared communities and places, to the upstream, culture, population and society. The links between these spheres of exclusion and connectedness are also discussed, to theorise an integrated framework for understanding the dynamics of social exclusion across dimensions of social action and along pathways of social processes.

The second part of the book presents a series of chapters, addressing areas of interest and knowledge gained through the experience and research of the authors. These chapters are presented so that, as readers, we come first to know the machinery of social exclusion and connectedness before coming to know the pathways towards exclusion, and finally come to know the excluded through their experience of exclusion and connection.

The third and final part of the book draws together the chapters thus far, finding points of congruence and dissension between spheres of action and applied areas of interest. In this short concluding part, we explore some of the implications for policy and practice, drawing on the chapters and research studies presented in Part 2 of the book. We also consider briefly a research agenda for the future.

A linguistic and cultural turn

At the outset, it is important to say something about the theoretical resources we use in our focus on social and cultural factors. Our understanding is that all social experiences and narratives about them are discursively constructed. This sets limits and constraints on the positions of exclusion, inclusion and connectedness that individuals and groups can take up. However individuals and groups are active, resistant agents in these processes and can shape the realm of discursive possibilities. Such a position recognises the importance of language, requiring a shift in view from language as a 'neutral tool, out there' to language as highly contingent: 'the fact that there is no way to step outside the various vocabularies we have employed and find a metavocabulary which somehow takes account of all possible vocabularies, all possible ways of judging and feeling' (Rorty 1989: xvi). We make sense of the world, our understandings of it, and our place in it, through language; our use of language creates, contests and recreates power, authority and legitimation.

Connected to this is the importance of a shift in view about identity, as Butler expresses it:

> the reconceptualisation of identity as an *effect*, that is, as *produced* or *generated*, opens up possibilities of 'agency' that are insidiously foreclosed by positions that take identity categories as foundational and fixed. For an identity to be an effect means that it is neither fatally determined nor fully artificial and arbitrary. That the *constituted* status of identity is misconstrued along these conflicting lines suggests the ways in which the feminist discourse on cultural construction remains trapped within the unnecessary binarism of free will and determinism. Construction is not opposed to agency; it is the necessary scene of agency, the very terms in which agency is articulated and becomes culturally intelligible.
>
> (Butler 1990: 147)

This notion of identity is taken up again in Chapter 1.2.

In terms of the analysis of social exclusion we present below, the foregoing should alert the reader that our analysis is based on a position of theoretical pluralism, which we argue is necessary to do justice to the complexity of the forces and relationships that shape individuals' and groups' experience of exclusion and being excluded. Suitable conceptualisations of notions of power are also required, and this is discussed later in Chapter 1.5.

Defining social exclusion

The notion of 'social exclusion' is a relatively new concept and is embedded in the economic, political and cultural/social structures of society; thus we need to be mindful of different interpretations of social exclusion, as well as of social inclusion and of social connectedness. It is a contested concept, with multiple meanings. We reserve discussion of social inclusion and connectedness for later, and here consider only social exclusion, Box 1.1 offers a short sketch of the history of use of the term, while Box 1.2 summarises some of the most often quoted definitions of social exclusion.

A number of different approaches to defining typologies that can assist in understanding social exclusion have been produced by various writers. Table 1.1 presents three rather different approaches. In the first, the approach focuses on defining different forms of exclusion; the second focuses on defining different types of participation, and the third on different types of exclusionary relationship.

Box 1.1. A brief history of social exclusion

- Term 'social exclusion' originated in France (Lenoir 1974) initially; French socialist politicians used social exclusion to refer to individuals who were not covered by the social security system.
- Over time the term broadened to cover other groups seen as excluded, for example, disaffected youth, the unemployed and the homeless. Reflected in Durkheimian philosophy, 'exclusion threatens society as a whole with the loss of collective values and destruction of the social fabric' – a 'deficiency in solidarity'. During the 1980s in France, the definition of social exclusion expanded to include the term *les éclus*, 'the pariahs of the nation', which gave rise to xenophobia, political attacks upon and restrictions on the rights of immigrants. In 1990s, exclusion included the issue of 'les banlieues', the deprived outer suburbs, which gave rise to combating 'urban exclusion' (Silver 1994).
- The terminology of social exclusion was adopted by the European Commission in its mandate to report, on a European-wide basis, about prevailing levels of poverty and unemployment. 'Social exclusion' was substituted for 'poverty' within European Union poverty programs from the 1990–4 programs onwards (Room 1995).
- There is a range of international European-based government agency programmes set up to ameliorate the impact of social exclusion: European Commission; World Bank; International Labour Organisation; United Nations Development Agency, which all have funded initiatives in place. These pan-national organisations tend to utilise the term in a broad sense to denote individuals and groups who are unable to secure adequate material (i.e. financial) and cultural capital (i.e. education and knowledge). In other words, social exclusion is used to describe those without the resources to access employment and educational networks.
- A moral discourse of 'social solidarity' saw 'The Third Way' emerge (Finlayson 1999; Jordan 2001; Levitas 2004), 'that would reconcile individual rights with state responsibility and socialist rejection of exploitation' (Silver 1994: 537). Social exclusion was adopted in Britain as a central notion in the UK Labour government's policies, post its 1997 election success. That year it established a government policy-making, multidisciplinary Social Exclusion Unit with the mission of tackling social exclusion.
- Mid-1990s, UK Economic and Social Research Council adopted 'social integration and exclusion' as one of its nine thematic priorities in social science research (Marsh and Mullins 1998: 759).

- 1997 – an Economic and Social Research Council funded 'Centre for the Analysis of Social Exclusion' was set up at the London School of Economics and Political Science.
- 2006 – Social Exclusion Knowledge Network (SEKN) set up, one of nine knowledge networks set up under WHO's Commission on Social Determinants of Health.
- February 2008, the final report of SEKN was produced (Popay *et al.* 2008).

Box 1.2. Frequently quoted definitions of social exclusion

- original French definition ('exclusion sociale'), as a 'rupture of social bonds' (European Foundation 1995, cited in de Haan 1998: 12)
- 'a shorthand term for what can happen when people or areas suffer from a combination of problems, such as unemployment, poor skills, low income, bad housing, high crime, poor health or lack of transport' (Social Exclusion Unit and Cabinet Office 2001: 2)
- 'inability to participate effectively in economic, social, political and cultural life, alienation and distance from the mainstream society' (Duffy 1995: 17)
- 'the dynamic process of being shut out ... from any of the social, economic, political and cultural systems which determine the social integration of a person in society' (Walker and Walker 1997: 8)
- 'sense of social isolation and segregation from the formal structures and institutions of the economy, society and the state' (Somerville 1998: 762)
- 'an individual is socially excluded if (a) he or she is geographically resident in a society but (b) for reasons beyond his or her control he or she cannot participate in the normal activities of citizens in that society and (c) he or she would like to participate' (Burchardt *et al.* 1999: 229)
- ESRC Centre for Analysis of Social Exclusion (Hills *et al.* 2002) suggests four dimensions: consumption – capacity to buy (now and future); production – participation in economically or socially valuable activities; political engagement – in local or national decision-making; social interaction with family, friends and community
- 'the continuous and gradual exclusion from full participation in the social, including material as well as symbolic, resources produced, supplied and exploited in a society for making a living, organizing a life and taking part in the development of a (hopefully better) future' (Steinert 2007a: 5)

- 'Social exclusion is a complex and multi-dimensional process. It involves the lack or denial of resources, rights, goods and services, and the inability to participate in the normal relationships and activities, available to the majority of people in society, whether in economic, social, cultural, or political arenas. It affects both the quality of life of individuals and the equity and cohesion of society as a whole' (Levitas *et al.* 2007: 9)
- 'Exclusion consists of dynamic, multi-dimensional processes driven by unequal power relationships interacting across four main dimensions – economic, political, social and cultural – and at different levels including individual, household, group, community, country and global levels. It results in a continuum of inclusion/exclusion characterised by unequal access to resources, capabilities and rights which leads to health inequalities' (Popay *et al.* 2008: 2)

In terms of particular disciplinary stances on social exclusion, Todman (2004) and Morgan *et al.* (2007) provide useful overviews of social exclusion (and its measurement) for social policy and mental health respectively. In examining Box 1.2, we can see conceptualisations of social exclusion as a state, a process or both. The definitions emphasise a varying list of factors that give rise to social exclusion which work together in such a way that often they end up reinforcing each other.

As a result of this inability to clearly define social exclusion, the term is often used in an indefinite way that is laden with economic, political and cultural nuances (Silver 1994). Further to this, attempts to establish a typology of social exclusion have been described as reductionist (Silver 1994). Social exclusion can be seen as a dynamic multi-dimensional process (Peace 2001; Steinert 2007a). As Bhalla and Lapeyre emphasise:

> Anglo-Saxon thinking is rooted in the Liberal paradigm and views society as a mass of atomized individuals in competition within the market place. Therefore, exclusion may reflect voluntary individual choices, patterns of interests or a contractual relationship between actors or 'distortions' to the system, such as discrimination, market failures and unenforced rights.
>
> (Bhalla and Lapeyre 1997: 415)

Importantly, no matter how social exclusion is conceptualised or defined, the notion often lends itself to the idea of deviance or non-conformity. This is particularly evident in current Australian welfare policy, for example, 'work for the dole', welfare to work, the Northern Territory indigenous policies including widespread alcohol bans, medical screening of all indigenous

Table 1.1 Typologies for understanding social exclusion

Typology label	Types	Source
Forms	• disengagement – lack of participation in social and community activities • service exclusion – lack of adequate access to key services when needed • economic exclusion – restricted access to economic resources and low economic capacity	Saunders *et al.* (2007)
Levels of participation	• survival, access to food, shelter, clothing etc • social relations, enhanced personal and familial reproduction • security, of means of survival and enhanced reproduction • production, autonomy of production of local, national and wider relevance • politics, organisation of infrastructure of production and reproduction • progress, take part in development of forces of production	Steinert (2007b)
Exclusionary relationships	• Horizontal vs. Vertical – horizontal exclusion excludes one from belonging to a group or network at the same level on the 'vertical ladder'. Vertical exclusion prevents individuals from climbing the vertical (social) ladder • Intentional vs. Unintentional – 'Intent' in social exclusion is typically linked to discrimination • Formal vs. Informal – while exclusion can be entrenched in institutions and legislation (e.g., the apartheid regime in South Africa), informal exclusion is more complex and challenging to confront, as it can involve traditional behaviours and patterns in society that may be difficult to detect • Multiple factor social exclusion – various forms of social exclusion can be experienced at once, for example (in the Nepali case) a Dalit woman from a remote area faces at least three causes of social exclusion, being a woman, being Dalit and being from a disadvantaged region • Reinforcing social exclusion – when groups are excluded from society, a domino effect can ensue (e.g. job loss leads to poverty leads to intergenerational disadvantage, etc.)	Renner *et al.* (2007)

children and quarantining welfare payments (Ring and Wenitong 2007). As Peace (2001) posits, using social exclusion as a policy framework runs the risk of structuring social policy negatively. Such a policy imposes power structures which perpetuate disparity and persistently work to undermine the empowerment attempts of the excluded (Alexander 2005). This is taken up and examined in several of the chapters in Part 2 including Cook's chapter (2.3) about women welfare recipients, and Taket, Foster and Cook's chapter (2.15) on silencing.

In their report on social exclusion produced for the WHO Commission on Social Determinants of Health, Popay *et al.* (2008) explored differences across the globe in discourses on social exclusion, as well as competing discourses operating within regions, pointing out how these draw on a range of different understandings of the term, linking these to the different national and international agencies active in the region, and stressing the importance of recognising this discursive diversity for policy and practice. Some of these issues are explored further in Part 2 in Lamaro's chapter about her work in South Africa (Chapter 2.13) and Renzaho's chapter about immigration (Chapter 2.9).

Social exclusion operates to prevent people from participating in the mainstream activities of society and accessing the standards of living enjoyed by the rest of society. At this point, it is useful to consider the distinction Viet-Wilson (1998) makes between weak and strong versions of social exclusion as they are expressed in policy discourse. Weak forms of social exclusion are based on a horizontal rather than a vertical model of social inequality. In vertical conceptions of inequality a continuum of positions is recognised, and the affluence and status of those higher up the continuum is dependent largely on the poverty and lack of status of those lower down. In the horizontal model, only a dichotomous distinction is recognised, one in which there are only the included and the marginalised; this renders the rich and powerful invisible, a small part of the large group of the included. Marmot's (2004) analysis points powerfully to the inadequacy of this horizontal model based on a simple dichotomy, and the material presented throughout this book also supports a more nuanced and complex understanding. The chapters in Part 2 by Pease on privilege (2.1) and Crisp on professional discretion (2.2) reflect on social exclusion from positions of power.

In the weaker versions of the discourse on social exclusion, the solutions to social exclusion lie in changing the characteristics of the excluded individuals in order to enhance their integration into society. In contrast the stronger forms of the discourse place emphasis on the role of those perpetuating the exclusion and aim to reduce their power. This is examined further in Pease's chapter (2.1).

The last three definitions in Box 1.2 are appealing to us for a number of different reasons. First they make explicit the idea that social exclusion is broader than poverty, broader than unemployment, encompassing issues of the denial of rights and lack of participation. Second they emphasise not only what social exclusion is, but what it gives rise to – its consequences, for individuals and for society, in both the short-run and over the longer term. These issues are taken up further in Part 2 in Savage and Carvill's chapter on carers (2.6), and Carey *et al.*'s chapter on childlessness (2.10). We incorporate elements of them into the framework presented below.

The framework we present for the analysis and understanding of processes of exclusion distinguishes three levels at which social exclusion operates: individual, community and society. In the three chapters that follow we explore these three levels in turn, before turning in Chapter 1.5 to exploring their dynamic interaction. Figure 1.1 depicts the framework.

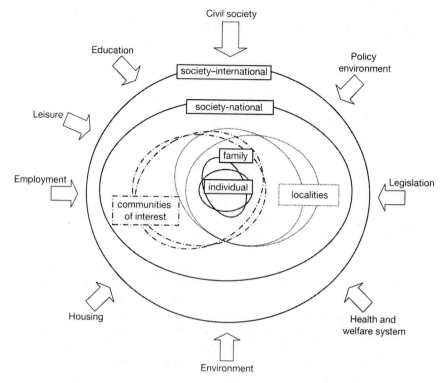

Key:
- Arrows – determinants of relations of exclusion – social, political, economic, etc. – whose effects are interactive, mediated discursively and non-discursively and operate variously at different levels, times, space and places
- Communities – of interest – bounded not by geography but by characteristics (hidden or visible) that constitute some shared interest. For any individual or family there will be multiple memberships, not all of which will be acknowledged or recognised at any particular time
- Localities – of life – living, working, leisure – 'communities defined by spaces and places

Figure 1.1 Framework for analysis of the production of relations of exclusion

In terms of the chapters that follow, our first level of focus is at the centre of Figure 1.1, where individuals and their experience of exclusion are considered. Next, in Chapter 1.3, we move on to the level of the community – considering here both communities defined by geography (localities on the figure) and those defined by interest. Chapter 1.4 considers the broader societal level. Finally in Chapter 1.5, we consider the links between the three different spheres of action.

1.2 The individual's experience

This chapter will focus on agency and the individual's experience of social exclusion. Whilst it is evident that the three levels are inextricably linked, the purpose of this section is to disentangle the experience of the socially excluded from the community and wider society in order to understand and explore the process of exclusion/inclusion for the individual. Social exclusion has a number of dimensions including the economic (concerned with income, employment and the labour market and the production of and/or access to goods and services including housing, health and education), the social (including participation in decision-making and opportunity for social participation), the political (civil and political rights and citizenship) and the spatial. Each of these can be related to the individual and the individual's relationship with the State and society (Bhalla and Lapeyre 1997).

An individual who is not socially excluded is not necessarily 'included'. Likewise, social inclusion does not imply social connectedness. Social connectedness refers to the relationships people have with others and the community (Ministry of Social Development 2007). The process of social connectedness is linked to social fabric and capital whereby multiple dimensions interact to create connectedness. Whilst an individual may be excluded, they may also experience strong social networks and connections. The mechanisms that influence social exclusion are linked to one's social capital. Social capital is a collective notion with its origins in individual behaviour, attitudes and predispositions (Brehm and Rahn 1997). Social capital facilitates individuals to gain (or lose) access to resources (Szreter and Woolcock 2004). It can be conceptualised as one of the building blocks that bond together individuals and communities. We return to this issue in Chapter 1.5.

Social exclusion of individuals is often based on assumptions of deviant behaviour and has often been conceptualised in terms of an 'underclass' which is confined to behavioural or biological representation of the lowest stratum of society (Martin 2004). The 'excluded' have traditionally included, but are not limited to, the unemployed, the poorly educated, the homeless, single parents, those with a disability, mental illness or substance use problem and criminals. Social exclusion has its roots in the labour market and economic wealth where an individual was either 'deserving' or 'undeserving'. The deserving were seen as those unable to support themselves such as the sick and elderly and the undeserving were those who in theory should have been able to support themselves. The latter group are assumed to be one or more of idle, lazy and criminal, and were subjected to punitive policies of control designed to force them into employment and self-sufficiency. This labelling can be seen throughout history and is evident in the English Poor Law Act of 1601 (Alcock 1997). However, over time, and as a result of welfare reform, the distinction of the excluded has shifted.

The individual's experience or process of exclusion may be voluntary or involuntary (Burchardt *et al.* 1999). The latter refers to the 'otherness' of individuals that experience disadvantage due to gender, age, ability, employment status, government policy or legislation, social norms and values and so forth. The voluntarily excluded refers to those individuals who choose to exclude or disconnect themselves from society. Burchardt *et al.* (1999) propose five dimensions by which to measure an individual's social exclusion: participation in activities of consumption, savings, production, politics and social. These are influenced by an individual's characteristics (e.g. health or education levels), life events, characteristics of the area in which one lives, and social, civil and political institutions of society. Chapter 2.14 by Barter-Godfrey and Taket returns to the issues of othering, marginalisation and pathways to exclusion in health.

The excluded are not a homogenous group; rather they are heterogeneous, crossing sociological lines, beliefs, cultures, political or religious affiliation and so forth. As such it is difficult and problematic to identify and describe the excluded in definitive terms. Individuals may experience exclusion in some aspects or times of their lives but in others feel complete inclusion. Whilst the critical realist approach allows for the empirical testing of theories of social exclusion, such an approach must first recognise that the language of exclusion and inclusion implies a dualism whereby one is either included or excluded. Such language is suggestive of people being excluded in relation to a particular variable or factor (O'Reilly 2005). Of course this raises the question of, if one is not excluded does that mean one is included? Rather than such a dualistic approach, exclusion should be seen as a continuum whereby individuals are positioned along a fluid continuum of absolute inclusion through to absolute exclusion, in terms of specific contexts. Thus, the positioning of any particular individual at a particular time in a particular context can be characterised as a multiple combination of inclusion and exclusion.

Individual agency operates at the micro-level in social exclusion and connection. The focus often is on the present experience of being socially excluded or connected and the behaviours, values, preferences and psychological factors associated with individual inclusion or exclusion. Status, class and consequence of life-choices are conceptualised as both the pathways to, and outcomes of, social exclusion. Bhalla and Lapeyre (1997) posit that individual citizens have the right to a certain basic standard of living and the right to participate in the major social and occupational institutions of the society.

Their arguments link individual behaviour, capacity for action and structural constraints and suggest that social exclusion occurs when individuals suffer from disadvantage and are unable to secure these social rights (Bhalla and Lapeyre 1997). Young (n.d.) posits that there are three basic positions in relation to agency. First, the victim blaming approach whereby the individual is 'blamed' for their own exclusion. Then there is the failure of the system, lack of employment opportunities, and thereby a lack of role models, which lead to social isolation. This is explored further by Stagnitti and Jennings in Chapter 2.8 in which they demonstrate how improving the reading skills of disadvantaged children lead to much greater levels of connectedness for whole families. The final position is that which sees the downsizing of industry, the stigmatisation of the workless, and the stereotyping of an underclass which is criminogenic, drug ridden with images which are frequently racialised and prejudiced as actively creating the excluded (Young n.d.). It is important to recognise that each of these three positions offers room for the exercise of individual agency; however there are often different moral understandings in operation in the different discourses attached to these positions (O'Reilly 2005).

> In the public policy arena a focus on specific different households can be linked with a labelling or pathologising approach that is often heavily value-laden and pejorative, even where there is a desire to identify disadvantage or diversity around gender, age, ethnicity or disability. It is all too short a step from identifying a group as one which faces problems, and is perceived as 'different', to presenting them as failures, deviant or culturally deficient.
>
> (Harrison 1998: 796)

Goffman provided the classic definition of stigma as a 'deeply discrediting attribute that globally devalues an individual' (Goffman 1963: 12). Negative health outcomes arise from different types of stigma, and fear of being stigmatised and feeling stigmatised lead to avoidance of potentially distressing situations, amounting to self-regulated exclusion. This provides a key mechanism by which social exclusion is created and maintained. Hall (2004) explores the social exclusion that many people with learning disabilities in Scotland experience. Despite their physical inclusion within communities in terms of housing and even employment, socially and culturally they narrate feeling unwelcomed and rejected, leading to them restricting their participation within certain spaces and places in their local communities of the non learning disabled, while at the same time seeking out and cultivating safe and welcoming spaces and places. Part 2 returns to the operation of stigma in processes of exclusion in Chapters 2.14 by Barter-Godfrey and Taket and 2.15 by Taket *et al.*, where we consider a number of different examples where stigma is implicated in inclusion or exclusion: those who experience intimate partner abuse, lesbians, gay men and bisexuals' use of the health service, women's participation in breast cancer screening and HIV positive women, while Chapter 2.11 by Nevill discusses the stigmatisation of older people.

Housing (Somerville 1998) presents one example where we can observe these processes of the creation of individuals belonging to a moral underclass (we discuss Levitas's work on the moral underclass discourse later in Chapter 1.4). Somerville examines social housing policy and highlights the cultural and behavioural individuality of two important groups in Britain; public housing tenants and the homeless. These groups are linked to unfavourable behaviours such as crime, substance use and teenage pregnancy (Watt and Jacobs 2000). The individual's behaviour is judged by societal norms and values and is viewed as deviant. These individuals or collectives of individuals are viewed as the 'problem' rather than as victims of the political, socio-economic and cultural structures which create the inequality. This inevitably leads to blaming the victim – those at the centre of what is perceived as deviant behaviour. Public housing is generally based on need and ability to wait; as such, the transient, young people, those with a disability or mental illness are often excluded from affordable, available housing. However, not being able to afford home ownership does not necessarily result in social exclusion, particularly if good quality rented accommodation can be secured. However, it also does not ensure inclusion (Somerville 1998). The labelling of individuals impacts on their housing access. Those seen as less deserving are channelled in to lower quality housing. We consider housing further in Chapter 2.4 by Henderson-Wilson.

A number of chapters in Part 2 illustrate similar processes at work in different domains for different types of individuals, for example, Chapter 2.3 by Cook looks at women's access to welfare benefits. Chapter 2.5 by Owens looks at people with disabilities and their access in a range of different domains. Chapter 2.11 by Nevill examines ageing, and Chapter 2.12 by Martin and Pallotta-Chiarolli considers bisexual young people in relation to substance abuse.

The notion of social exclusion is gendered in that those who hold roles such as mothers and carers are judged by society as not participating in the labour market or contributing to society, suggesting little value is placed on these roles. Cook and Marjoribanks' (2005) work suggests that the current welfare policies in Australia are closely aligned with the moral underclass discourse. This is particularly evident in regard to low-income mothers who feel penalised by factors outside their control which impact on their ability to contribute to the labour market (Cook and Marjoribanks 2005). Such welfare agendas demonstrating the labelling of individuals at a policy level based on their circumstance can induce a victim blaming approach and the connotations of such labelling can be part of the process by which they are excluded, rather than the circumstances themselves. Two particular examples discussed in Part 2 are Cook's chapter about female welfare recipients (Chapter 2.3) and Carey *et al.*'s chapter about childless women (Chapter 2.10).

The moral underclass discourse suggests that social exclusion of individuals occurs as a process which is influenced by what is viewed deviant or immoral. Sexuality is one such area where individuals have been socially excluded from 'mainstream' society based on their sexual behaviour. For example, non-heterosexuality has historically been viewed as immoral, particularly by church groups. As a result individuals are excluded from full civic participation (Kitchin and Lysaght 2004). From this perspective it is clear that social exclusion at the individual level is not just associated with the labour markets. It is influenced by societal beliefs and structures which act to 'exclude' individuals based on personal characteristics. Similar patterns can be seen in regard to culture and ethnicity. Kabeer (2006) explores this area in terms of what she calls the challenge of durable inequality in the development of Asian social protection policies, identifying that there are significant forms of persistent disadvantage not fully captured by economic approaches or measurements in some Asian cultures. These revolve around aspects related to identity, and reflect the cultural devaluation of people based on who they are, or rather, who or what they are perceived to be. This may relate to membership of a particular group of people, who acknowledge their commonality, have shared beliefs and values and act in collective ways. Caste, ethnicity and religion are examples of such group identities. Alternatively, the identities may relate to categories of people defined on the basis of some shared, devalued or stigmatised characteristic. Street children, people with leprosy or AIDS and undocumented migrants are examples of such socially excluded categories. Part 2 takes up these issues in Chapters 2.12 in relation to sexuality, and 2.9 and 2.15 in relation to ethnicity as well as HIV positive status.

Steinert and Pilgram (2007) present a fascinating insight into cross-European diversity in individuals' understandings and experience of exclusion. Their study, carried out in eight European cities with very diverse welfare regimes, is based on respondent-centred interviews with 1,281 individuals yielding 3,291 narratives about episodes of exclusion. The study is an excellent example of the value of comparative research across different welfare systems and social policy contexts. For example, Rönneling and Gabàs i Gasa (2007) explore how the narratives of the Swedish and Spanish informants differ according to the normative assumptions present about the welfare system and its operation. The Swedish respondents expected a wide scope and efficient functioning of the welfare system – where these expectations were not fulfilled, frustration and indignation towards the system were expressed. In contrast, amongst the Spanish respondents expressions of indignation were rare, the level of expectation and scope was different, and the focus of the narratives was on the alternative ways of coping. As the authors point out however, we do not know to what extent, or if at all, non-state resources play a role in coping strategies in Sweden; we only learn that the respondents placed more emphasis on public resources.

Having considered briefly social exclusion at the level of the individual, we next turn our attention to the level of the community.

1.3 Social exclusion and community

The English satirical novelist Sue Townsend has written of a nation in which intentional communities for the socially excluded was government policy:

> In a desperate attempt to be seen to be 'doing something' about crime and social disorder, the Government's Department of Liveability embarked on a bold program to convert the satellite council estates into Exclusion Zones, where the criminal, the antisocial, the inadequate, the feckless, the agitators, the disgraced professionals, the stupid, the drug-addicted and the morbidly obese lived cheek by jowl.
>
> (Townsend 2006: 11–12)

One of the exclusion zones in this fictional world was the 'Flowers Exclusion Zone' (FEZ), owned by multi-millionaire Arthur Grice, whose private police force enforced the numerous restrictions on residents as well as continuously monitoring every aspect of their existence:

> A twenty-foot-high metal fence topped with razor wire and CCTV cameras formed the boundary between the back gardens of Hell Close and the outside world. At the only entrance to the FEZ, on a triangular piece of muddy ground, squatted a series of interconnected Portakabins, housing the Grice Security Police. The residents of the zone were required to wear an ankle tag and carry an identity card at all times. Their movements were followed by the security police on a bank of CCTV screens, installed in one of the Portakabins. ...
>
> There were many prohibitions and restrictions imposed on the residents of the FEZ. A strict curfew had to be adhered to; residents must be inside their homes from 10 p.m. until 7 a.m. at weekends. During the week they must be inside their houses from 9.30 p.m. Residents were not allowed to leave the estate. All correspondence, both in and out of the Exclusion Zone, was read and censored as appropriate. The telephone system did not extend to the outside world. There were only two free-to-view channels, the Advertising Channel, which showed a few programs now and

then, and the Government News Channel, which, unsurprisingly, had a perceptible bias in favour of the Government.

(Townsend 2006: 12–13)

Although Townsend has produced a caricature of a community which is almost entirely comprised of individuals who are at risk of social exclusion, and which is cut off from the wider world, it nevertheless reflects the thinking underpinning many policy and practice interventions to reduce social exclusion. Policy initiatives regularly target local communities on the basis of having high numbers of individuals who have low incomes and/or are members of an ethnic minority or some other factor which suggests social exclusion is likely (Geddes 2000; Watt and Jacobs 2000; Andersen and van Kempen 2003; Judge and Bauld 2006). This is despite the claims that socially excluded individuals are more likely to live outside areas where social exclusion is readily recognised (Commins 2004). For example, while rural environments are increasingly being packaged as 'consumption products' sold to urban populations to meet their leisure needs, it is important however not to regard rural areas as idyllic or problem-free as Maidment and Macfarlane note in Chapter 2.7. Despite the fact that images of poverty and social exclusion may not be as readily apparent as on some urban housing estates, life for many rural dwellers is not the romantic dream encapsulated in picture postcards (Commins 2004) and social exclusion is a very real issue despite contentions that it tends to be a problem only for urban communities (Mullins *et al.* 2001; Power and Wilson 2000).

While recognising that there are communities which include high numbers of individuals who are socially excluded from the wider society, it is important to recognise two other ways in which notions of community and social exclusion interact. The first of these concerns exclusion of individuals or groups within a community. The second concerns the exclusion of communities from full participation in the wider society.

Exclusion within communities

In any community, individuals who perceive they are outside societal norms, for example as a result of gender, sexual orientation, race and ethnicity, disability or illness, religion or political views, may feel alienated from both the wider community and/or from their own bodies (Cheng 2006). While who is excluded may be formally denoted and maintained by policies and procedures of government and/or other public authorities (Lukes 1997) or outspoken lobby groups (Kitchin and Lysaght 2004), the criteria by which individuals come to experience exclusion may not be readily articulated. Exclusion can even occur despite specific intentions aimed at ensuring inclusion (Kitchin 1998; Kitchin *et al.* 1998). Irrespective of how exclusion occurs, perceptions of being excluded can readily lead to the situation whereby 'much effort will be expended not to be among the losers, whether in terms of finance, health, reputation or whatever' (Alison 2003: 29–30). This process can begin in childhood. Even though they may not know why they are excluded, children readily learn of their excluded status (Richardson and Le Grand 2002).

As to who is excluded, this can vary considerably between communities, but those most at risk of exclusion are those with limited opportunities for financial advancement, newcomers to a community and persons who transgress the ideologies or dominant moral code of a community. The likelihood of exclusion is enhanced, the more categories an individual or group falls into. For instance, in many countries, foreigners are marginalised in respect of their place in the labour market and in other areas of social and cultural participation (Somerville 1998). However, there can be exceptions to these theories, and in some circumstances those one might expect to be excluded are embraced by a community. For example, it has been suggested that the predominantly Catholic Polish migrants have been well accepted in Spain, as many brought with them forms of religious practice and commitment which had in previous generations been widespread among the Spanish, and of which contemporary Spaniards had fond memories (Goicoechea 2005).

Historically, length of residence, of either the individual or their family, has frequently been regarded as a predictor of a sense of belonging to a particular community. The theory is that those who are long-established within a community are more likely to be more involved both in community activities and have larger social networks (Sampson 1991). However, in an era in which neighbourhoods are increasingly being packaged as products for consumption (Forrest and Kearns 2001), understandings of inclusion and exclusion based on length of tenure are being overturned. Indeed it has been suggested that:

> the sense of place, its meaning and people's attachment to a locality or neighbourhood is no longer constructed through historical attachments or long residence, leading to an 'authentic' attachment to place, but instead is constructed out of mobility, global interconnections and, especially for the middle classes, a deliberate decision to live there and identify with that place.
>
> (McDowell *et al.* 2006: 2164)

Conversely, it has been proposed that 'mobility is now understood to be a freedom bought by money and education. Remaining in the same place symbolizes a lack of choice that is the lot of the poor, the elderly, and people with disabilities' (Sheldrake 2001: 48). For young people whose access to education and employment opportunities may be restricted as a result of living in a rural area, leaving may be perceived as the only viable option (Alston and Kent 2003).

The extent to which an individual or group feels included or excluded in a particular community may differ substantially from the extent to which they feel accepted by the wider society. Members of minority groups are much more likely to become involved in their community when they are aligned with one of the dominant groups within that community (Portnoy and Berry

1997). Participation can also be affected by the physical infrastructure such as adequate community facilities (Kitchin 1998; Kitchin and Law 2001) or transport systems (Barrett *et al.* 2003). While an absence of these can make it difficult for disabled people to venture outside the home at any time, poor infrastructure can result in partial exclusion of other members of the community. For example, in many places women are encouraged not to use public transport or walk alone at night, particularly in areas which are unlit. Those who do so, are made to feel that it is their own fault if they are attacked or abused in such circumstances (Hodgson and Turner 2003).

In an era when an increasing number of life functions, including banking, shopping, work, leisure activities and communication, can all be transacted online, it is sometimes proposed that for individuals who feel alienated from their geographical community, the internet is a safe place to connect with like others on issues, when they would not feel safe to do so in their own community (Cheng 2006). The internet has also opened up opportunities for non-dominant perspectives to be shared more widely:

> Might this be a way to build virtual community at a time of increasing fragmentation? Might it be a medium that would allow the deaf to far more effectively engage in a conversation whose words need to be seen, and from which they experience exclusion by the hearing?
>
> (Simmonds 2000: 264)

While, undoubtedly, the internet has much potential for reducing feelings of isolation of individuals who experience exclusion, it is not a panacea to the effects of exclusion within communities. Notwithstanding debates as to the necessity for some degree of 'enfleshed encounters' (Simmonds 2000: 264), the financial costs involved may be beyond those of many individuals who experience marginalisation within their communities. Furthermore, access to high-speed internet connections which are increasingly necessary to use many internet-based services, are not always available, particularly in rural communities, as Maidment and Macfarlane note in Chapter 2.7.

Excluded communities

When substantial numbers of excluded individuals live in a community, stigmatisation of the entire community may result. In communities which are stigmatised on the basis of seemingly high crime rates or perceptions that socially unacceptable behaviours flourish, such as illegal drug use, teenage pregnancies, high unemployment and/or truancy from schools, discourses about a moral underclass are readily transformed from being a debate about some members of a community to imputing beliefs about all members of the community (Watt and Jacobs 2000). Consequently, living in a stigmatised community can hinder one's prospects of participation in employment or other opportunities afforded to those who live in neighbouring communities which are viewed more favourably by outsiders (Richardson and Le Grand 2002). Not surprisingly, there are frequently many individuals and families who will seek to move from what they experience as excluded communities to live in what they perceive to be better neighbourhoods or communities. However, there will also be families who make a deliberate choice to live in stigmatised neighbourhoods, on the basis that housing prices are substantially lower, which might result in an overall higher standard of living (Buck 2001).

Communities with a high level of social capital are more likely to receive effective and efficient services which benefit all members of the community (Narayan and Pritchett 1999). This can occur even in communities which on many other indicators would be ranked as highly marginalised. An example of such a community is Fitzroy in the inner suburbs of Melbourne. In the 1940s, it was regarded as the 'worst slum in Melbourne', but efforts from a local welfare agency in partnership with the local community enabled the poor housing conditions to be filmed and shown to the relevant politicians, as well as protests against unfair laws for tenants and landlords being organised which also received attention outside the local community. These actions resulted not only in the clearance of the slums but in a major change in the provision of public housing in the state of Victoria (Brotherhood of St Laurence n.d.). Several decades later when the Fitzroy community faced the closure of its swimming pool in 1994, a high profile media campaign, including a 'pool party' attended by 4,000 people in the empty swimming pool which was addressed by community members with high media profiles, was credited with saving this community facility (Crisp 2000).

Communities which are outside the viewpoint of policy makers are particularly at risk of exclusion. In particular, it has frequently been argued that urban policy makers tend not to take into account the perspectives of rural stakeholders in their determinations. For example,

> Development policy and planning have historically revolved around quests for large successes. Policy makers, usually located in urban centres, take a bird's-eye view of nations or regions and set out to create change at a macro scale, with significant impacts – through a major new industry, or a large and visible infrastructure project, or public policies based on utilitarian principles. Yet over time, it has become increasingly obvious that macro-scale successes can only be micro-scale disasters. At the same time as a nation or a region overall may reap benefits, particular communities and groups can be suffering losses: of land, livelihoods, opportunities, or autonomy. And, while the macro-statistics may indicate more production, more infrastructure, better health and housing, more access to employment and education, or more services – that is, successful development – significant pockets of the population may find themselves isolated from these benefits.
>
> (Eversole and Martin 2005: 176)

An example of this occurring is that in a time of severe drought in much of Australia, decisions were often being made by urban bureaucrats as to whether farm families in an area were eligible to seek financial assistance. In regions where farmers received some drought compensation payments, this not only benefited farming families but also the wider community through the injection of money into local economies. In areas in which farmers did not receive these payments, but considered their circumstances to be similar to their peers in other areas who did benefit from the seemingly discretionary decisions made from afar, the impact on the community could be substantial (Alston 2005).

In order to get their views heard by urban policy makers, rural communities may have to be pro-active, rather than wait for someone to come and consult them. The skills and capacities of both individuals and organisations are crucial for enhancing the participation of local communities in regional decision-making, as well as providing a regional voice into statewide or national decision-making processes (Head 2005). This in turn may require specific training to be designed for community members, if partnerships between local communities and outside providers of services are to be effective (Hull 2006).

1.4 Social exclusion at the societal level

Social exclusion theories of population and society have evolved over time, and definitions of social exclusion are closely linked to the ways social integration at the societal level have been defined and theorised. Silver (1994) distinguished three paradigms describing social exclusion, and our discussion of these draws on her paper and Saraceno's (2001) commentary on it: solidarity, specialisation and monopoly.

The first of these paradigms, the solidarity paradigm, was dominant in France, where exclusion was seen as a deficiency of solidarity (having both cultural and moral connotations) within society rather than an economic or political phenomenon. The paradigm can be traced to French republican notions of solidarity. The solidarity paradigm is aligned with Levitas' (1998) social integrationist discourse.

The second paradigm, specialisation, is Anglo-American in origin and is based on liberal-individualism. Here exclusion results from the operation of discrimination and inability to overcome various different types of barriers. There is a shared understanding of inclusion as occurring mainly through paid work so that it is necessary 'to make work pay', however the British tradition recognises that social exclusion also involves access to social rights. This paradigm is aligned with Levitas' (1998) moral underclass discourse. Fear of a permanent underclass exists, suggesting the poor may be permanently excluded. Criticism has been directed to this line of thinking, arguing it is important to differentiate between groups who go through transient phases of poverty compared with those who are permanently poor or excluded.

The third paradigm, the monopoly or social closure paradigm stems from Weberian work in the antipositivist tradition, and is prevalent in many northern European countries. This paradigm foregrounds power relations, pointing to powerful class and status groups, which have distinct social and cultural identities as well as institutions, and which use social closure to restrict the access of other groups to different types of valued resources, including good jobs, good benefits, education, urban locations, valued patterns of consumption, etc. This paradigm is also aligned with Levitas' (1998) redistributive discourse. In examining this paradigm, Saraceno (2001: 8) commented that this 'points to the material and cultural/symbolic privileges of the insiders as the cause of the exclusion of outsiders'.

Implicit in the foregoing discussion is an emphasis on understanding exclusion in terms of processes (rather than as a state) and further, understanding these processes as particularly dynamic. This means, in understanding these processes we need to identify both the factors affecting the processes of exclusion as well as the particular groups experiencing exclusion.

Room and Britton (2006) draw attention to the dynamics of social exclusion in terms of interactions between different levels, changing circumstances at the level of households are mediated by processes at the institutional level. As they identify, organisations and institutions whose activities shape household fates do so in ways that are socially unequal. Households that are already disadvantaged are in general less able to shape these institutional priorities and processes. More serious perhaps, is that under some circumstances, factors can progressively reinforce each other to such an extent that some households are sent along catastrophic downward trajectories, while the institutions that support them are progressively degraded. The dramatic effects of negative feedback loops in the system are well illustrated in Wilson's (1987) analysis of the US urban ghetto.

Citizenship is an important form of participation at the macro, state level, and lack of or ineligibility for citizenship is a form of social exclusion, a form for which examples abound. Berman and Phillips (2000) discuss examples such as where children of foreign parents born in Austria do not automatically gain citizenship, and consequently suffer restricted access to education and employment. Other sources of exclusion at the state or national level can be found in various forms of discriminatory legislation that establishes different levels of rights for different population groups. One example with far-reaching consequences is the status and rights of indigenous peoples. The extent to which the rights of indigenous peoples have been compromised varies across the globe, and their exclusion has often been supported by legislation which has taken a long time to overturn as discriminatory (Stavenhagen 2005). Within Australia, exclusion of indigenous people has also been maintained through official discourses such as law, government reports, policy and program objectives, media commentary and scholarship, as Havemann (2005) illustrates in his analysis of the origins of and the consequences of exclusion still manifest in the placelessness of Australia's indigenous people. He identifies a history of some steps towards reconciliation, but also a clear statement of where these fall short. Since his analysis, further positive steps, including Kevin Rudd's historic apology have taken place, but these fall far short of removing the exclusionary processes that continue to saturate Australian federal and state institutions and their policies.

Humpage (2006), considering the case of the Maori in New Zealand, illustrates the need for societies containing indigenous peoples to develop policy that reflects their own socio-political circumstances, rather than simply adopt policy discourses that are popular internationally. She explores how the goal of an 'inclusive society', which has framed New Zealand social policy since 1999, promotes an equal opportunity approach that sits in tension with the specific needs and rights of Maori as indigenous peoples and partners in the 1840 Treaty of Waitangi. The New Zealand 'Closing the Gaps' strategy of the 1990s stressed that the socio-economic exclusion of Maori set them apart from other New Zealand citizens. In contrast, the foreshore and seabed policy framed Maori as the same as other New Zealanders; they deserved the right to enjoy full protection of the seabed and foreshore but only under an equal citizenship approach, not a Treaty rights framework. The social exclusion/ inclusion discourse could not conceive of rights additional to citizenship, such as indigenous and Treaty rights. In addition, despite promising to tackle the 'root causes' of exclusion through social investment, the Labour-coalition government used this discourse to shift away from endorsing a structural explanation for Maori socio-economic exclusion and from accepting that a shift in power between the state and Maori is necessary for the latter to be included.

Takács (2006) reviews a wide range of European research which demonstrates the vulnerability of lesbian, gay, bisexual and transgender youth in EU member states to social exclusion in most aspects of their lives, as was also demonstrated by Heaphy and Yip (2006) in their work on older lesbians and gay men.

Exclusion has a geographic dimension, as participation in society depends on proximity, mobility, networks and location. Even being located in a lower socio-economic environment may precipitate discrimination at many levels Klasen (n.d.). Khakee *et al.* (1999) demonstrates the extent to which minority and migrant groups have been excluded from the process of urban renewal in various European contexts. Changes in the employment sphere and transformation in the relationships between waged work, gender and class in McDowell's (2000) study have resulted in a situation where, in terms of education and employment, young men in particular are falling behind and into economic exclusion. This is the case, in the USA, for African-American males (Sanchez-Jankowski 1999; Johnson *et al.* 2000), but also for migrant groups in European cities (Khakee *et al.* 1999).

Kenna (2007) reports a study of the contribution of master planned estates to polarisation in the urban landscape. Her research analysed the intentions, imagery and outcomes of a specific master planned estate in suburban Sydney. The developers and place marketers played a key role in the construction of an image of an exclusive and prestigious estate for white nuclear families. This ultimately superseded some of the more socially inclusive planning objectives for the area. Her conclusion was that there is an explicit connection between intentions and imagery, which encourages socio-spatial polarisation.

Selwyn (2002) viewed the UK's use of information and communication technology (ICT) as a social inclusion strategy as shifting attention from the real causes of social exclusion. Nevertheless, Van Winden (2001) reports the results of a study into the beneficial contributions of ICTs in three European cities (Manchester, Rotterdam and The Hague) on participation in social networks, local decision making and political processes and economic life. No convincing evidence was found that social networks of excluded groups were being strengthened; nor were there any signs of increased political participation and influence of deprived groups. However, for the economic dimension of exclusion, there were some indications that ICT policy may lead to reintegration in the economic system. Van Winden advances a number of reasons why the results were not as favourable as hoped, including insufficient time for full adoption, and concludes that there is a role for ICT in the support of social inclusion policy, and this depends upon, among other things, the capacity of urban management to align the application of ICT with other social inclusion policies.

Fairclough's interesting analysis of the language used by New Labour in Britain yields the central conclusion that: 'In the language of New Labour social exclusion is an outcome rather than a process – it is a condition people are in rather than something that is done to them' (Fairclough 2000: 54). Hence the conception of social exclusion drawn on is the weakest of the weak versions. Byrne's own analysis of the UK concludes that 'the character of UK "anti-exclusion" policies and the form of understanding of social exclusion that informs them actually contributes to the development of an excluding post-industrial capitalism based on poor work for many and insecurity for most' (Byrne 2005: 1). His further analysis focused on the US, France and Germany leads him to conclude that 'advanced industrialised societies are converging on a norm of social politics organized around a flexible labour market and structural social exclusion'. In other words, social exclusion is something required by advanced market capitalism for its functioning. As Finlayson (1999) points out, others, like Giddens (1998), are not convinced that capitalism has structural tendencies towards exclusion and oppression. It was to Giddens' views that the UK Labour government under Tony Blair looked for the theoretical underpinning of its view on the third way and its policy stance on social exclusion.

Byrne's analysis further identifies how the weak usage of social exclusion, and Fairclough's adjectival as opposed to verb form use of the expression, positions exclusion as a condition rather than a process. This is exceptionally important in helping construct the range of possible social politics in post-industrial societies and in stifling challenges to the view of market capitalism is the only possible form of future social arrangement.

Note however that Byrne's analysis, although it calls for a recognition of a strong form of social exclusion (defined as that form that emphasises the role of those who help constitute the relations of excluding) and aims for solutions that reduce the powers of exclusion, is of a limited nature in that it concentrates on social exclusion as economic exploitation (a political economic analysis) and not as domination. So that for Byrne, the question of exclusion on the basis of gender, sexuality, race, etc., although he recognises all as being valid – referring to this as 'excluded identities' – is not what is dealt with in the current debate on social exclusion. This is a limitation of his analysis – in that he ignores the multiple forms of social exclusion that *are* alluded to in discussion, for example, in regeneration circles at the local level in non-political circles (Raco 2002), and his field of analysis is restricted to the economic sector within the national policy arena. So while his analysis is extremely important, in this book we want to turn the main focus of our attention to the other sectors in society, and the different spheres of action.

1.5 Social exclusion and the threads between the spheres

We have proposed that social exclusion and connection can be considered in three broad spheres of action: individual agency, community and society. Our approach has similarities to that of Gallie (2004), who presents his ideas on social isolation by describing three major spheres of sociability: the primary (micro) sphere involving connection to immediate family and household residents; the secondary (meso) sphere regarding interactions with people outside the household, and the tertiary (macro) sphere involving participation in external structures and the broader environment. There are also resonances with three levels (biographical, life-world and structural) used in Steinert and Pilgram (2007). Our approach also has strong similarities with the relational framework described in Abrams and Christian (2007), whose analysis distinguishes four different elements: the actors in an exclusion relationship (sources and targets of exclusion), the relationship context (across a series of levels from intrapersonal through to societal and trans-national), the modes/forms of exclusion (ideological/moral, representational, categorical, physical, communicative) and the dynamics of the exclusion relationship (the why and when exclusion happens). Where our emphasis differs, however, is on its focus on the interactions between the different elements in the system that create and recreate exclusionary relationships.

We have seen similar themes occurring within these different spheres, such as deprivation as individual poverty, underserved communities and population inequities of resource allocation or availability; and isolation as family breakdown, fractured communities and disengaged populations. Therefore in order to understand the dynamics of exclusion and connection across different layers of human action and interaction, it is important to reflect on how these concentric spheres influence each other and the common pathways that run through them. The following section discusses the 'threads' that extend between individuals, communities and populations.

The threads that permeate our daily spheres of activity can be the 'snakes and ladders' of disadvantage, being the dynamic processes and pathways to exclusion and inclusion/connectedness. For social exclusion, these threads can be the labour market, low income, unemployment, education, ill health, housing, transport, crime and fear of crime, language, mobility, social policies and social capital (Buchanan 2007). Issues relating to housing policy are considered in Chapter 2.4 by Henderson-Wilson, education policy by Stagnitti and Jennings in Chapter 2.8, and health policy by Barter-Godfrey and Taket in Chapter 2.14.

For inclusion/connectedness, these threads act as the ladders of opportunity and access, acceptance, identity and citizenship (Sullivan 2002). Owens' Chapter 2.5 considers the specific case of access and people with disabilities, while Stagnitti and Jennings, in Chapter 2.8 look at the role of a pre-school reading preparation program on social inclusion of marginalised families. These threads can be the outcomes, structures, processes and barriers that lead to inclusion and exclusion, and can affect many domains within everyday life, such as health, public order, economic stability and debt, integration and neighbourhood decline/renewal (Welshman 2006a, 2006b).

However, these barriers and opportunities are not evenly distributed throughout a society; social exclusion often reflects unfair economic, power and class structures (Labonte 2004). Burdens of social exclusion may be geographic, demographic or social; and include age, ethnicity, gender, class, sexuality, disability, citizenship and socio-economic ones (Train *et al.* 2000; Jarman 2001). The comprehensive report of the WHO Commission on the Social Determinants of Health, chaired by Michael Marmot (CSDH 2008) makes this, and the links to consequent burdens of ill-health and lack of wellbeing, abundantly clear. There are particular challenges for different groups. Nevill, in Chapter 2.11, looks at the case of older people, while Martin and Pallotta-Chiarolli (Chapter 2.12) examine the complex issues involved in bisexual young people, marginalisation and mental health in relation to substance abuse. These life chances, rather than life choices, represent threads of burden that are inequitably concentrated in vulnerable, disempowered, deprived and poor parts of a society, geographically and socially. Social justice calls for action to achieve the absence or alleviation of these experiences and social biases that leave people 'captive, bound and double-ironed' (Dickens 1843), based on three principles of social justice: equal rights to basic liberties, equality of opportunity, and the balance of inequalities to favour the least advantaged (Lutz 2002; Rawls 1971). In this way, exclusion and connectedness are not necessarily converse ideas, but are embedded within broader principles of justice, equity and fairness. It is with the idea of embeddedness that we next consider our threads as the connections within and between societies.

Social capital, contested concept though it is, represents the sticky threads that glue us together and is a useful heuristic to draw links between the micro, meso and macro levels of disadvantage and our three spheres of action (Cattell 2004; Schuller *et al.* 2000). It has long philosophical roots, but was revived as a concept in the last two decades of the twentieth century, with structures, functions and resources being important dimensions in understanding the role of connections in social exclusion and inclusion (Morrow 2001; Patulny and Svendsen 2007).

Following Putnam's model, bonding social capital is 'social glue', analogous to Marx's bounded solidarity and Durkheim's mechanical solidarity, where social cohesion is shared by people with similarities, which can range from similar ideals and objectives, similar activities or mutual social relationships. Bridging capital is 'social oil' and may be parallel to Marx's aggregate social capital and Durkheim's organic solidarity, as a source of social cohesion through the networks, cooperation, reliance and reciprocity between different groups and strata in civic society (see Marx 1894; Durkheim 1893; Putnam 1993, 2000; Aldridge *et al.* 2002; Wilson 2006). Whereas these bonding and bridging forms of social capital have different social *functions* for the common good and civic resources, earlier models emphasised civic resource *structures* and accessing individualised benefits.

Bourdieu describes social capital as first the social relationships that facilitate individual access to resources, and second the proliferation and quality of resources, so that social capital requires civic investment to develop social capital structures, which cumulatively foster other forms of capital, such as economic, cultural and human capital, as the outcome of social action and connection (see Bourdieu 1985, 1986). Social capital is therefore a comment on both the prevalence of sticky threads within a community or population, and also, on whether or not these threads permeate into the sphere of a particular individual.

Complementary to these two approaches, Halpern's model combines components, functions and levels. Components include networks, norms and sanctions. Functions draw on principles of bridging and bonding capital, as well as linking capital that bridges between asymmetric power relationships, and levels of analysis and action cover micro-level close family and friends, meso-level communities and associations and the macro, national level (Halpern 2005). In this way, there are top-down threads, structures and sanctions imposed through population processes surrounding individual 'hubs', coupled with bottom-up threads and functional norms generated within communities. This relatively broader 'Catherine wheel' conceptualisation of social capital is useful for capturing the complexities of social factors and emphasising the embeddedness of capital and cohesion processes.

Models of social capital, in particular Halpern's but also its antecedents, can be helpful to draw out and explain the intuitive threads running through social spheres and experiences, moving beyond the more categorical approaches to threads as barriers, ladders and shackles. Unlike principles of equity and access, social capital is not necessarily a benign process and may be both inclusive and exclusive; mutuality and affiliation can reinforce inequalities, concentrate power without mandate and quango community norms, including criminality and exclusion (Lin 2001; Portes 1998). Bonding capital in particular may increase exclusion by protecting the boundaries of the in-group and norms of participation (Piachaud 2002; Leonard 2004). Bourdieu's approach to social capital (Bourdieu 1985, 1986) recognises the inherent value of conflict and power-negotiation in developing social capital, trust and community-established advancement, and celebrates differences within populations, even when that leads to competition or difference in ideals.

Like Foucault's concept of 'technologies of power' (Foucault 1978), some of the connecting threads between individuals and groups are forms of control, normalisation and adherence. Marginalisation can therefore be the outcome of a mismatch between the norms and aspirations communicated through threads of social power and control, and the individual's identification with or ability to achieve those expectations. A culture of high-expectation can be empowering for those who can achieve but can also foster alienation when fulfilment of commonly held aspirations is not attainable in all communities (Young 1998) where the threads of social desirability are prevalent and idealised, but do not reach equitably into communities and do not reach far enough into individuals' spheres. In this way, exclusion is not merely the absence of inclusion; connections may reinforce alienation when they are irreconcilable with other dimensions of an individuals' reality whilst gaps in economic and social connections amplify other exclusionary processes.

Other aspects of Foucault's theoretisation of power are also important to us here. The threads winding between the spheres from individual up through to societal level point to the importance of a critical scrutiny of the construction of the subject/identity and the operation of power, as the point of its operation is also the point at which resistance is/can be sited (or sighted). Three of Foucault's methodological precautions in looking at power are of particular pertinence here: to examine domination and the material operators of power; to study 'power at the point where its intention ... is completely invested in its real and effective practices' (Foucault 1976: 97); to analyse power as something that circulates, recognising that 'individuals ... are always in the position of simultaneously undergoing and exercising ... power. They are not only its inert or consenting target; they are always also the elements of its articulation. In other words, individuals are the vehicles of power, not its points of application' (Foucault 1976: 98).

Following Gordon's discussion of Foucault (Gordon 1980), we argue that our understanding of the constructed nature of subjects/identity requires an exploration of the historical conditions of possibility of present social/human science in relation to (against and with) the exploration of a vast array of practices and techniques, both discursive and non-discursive, that contribute to the disciplining, surveillance, administration and formation of groupings of individuals, at levels from the smallest unit of the individual subject, through the family through communities to national and supra-national populations. It also requires the recognition that this is not a strictly hierarchical structure.

Communities of interest can constitute themselves across a variety of different levels, and the internet has enabled the mobilisation of such communities to achieve social and political goals. A classic example is provided by its use in late June 1999, to provide a networked form of organisation of the protests/carnivals that took place in cities across the globe on 18 June 1999, timed to coincide with the opening of the G8 summit in Cologne. A campaign to cancel Third World debt was the touchstone but the aims of the day were far wider. Organised by loose networks of small groups and individuals, within internet-based communication of information, a wide variety of action took place – electronic forms of protest (a virtual sit-in), as well as actions requiring physical presence; central co-ordination or direction were not apparent. Web sites contained links to 43 different country sites, alternative sites were made available for when the traffic on others became too great. This form of organising was heralded in some quarters as posing a unique challenge to the authorities in terms of attempting to respond. Reports presented a mixture of predominantly carnival, with some violence against property (on the part of the demonstrators) and against people and property (on the part of the police and authorities). The events are documented still at various places across the internet, see http://www.urban75.org/j18/index.html (last accessed 22 November 2008) for example.

There is also a need to set aside the polarisation of the subject-object relationship which privileges subjectivity as the form of moral autonomy, in favour of a conception of domination as able to take the form of a subjectification as well as of an objectification; and second, the rejection of the assumption that domination falsifies the essence of human subjectivity, and the assertion that power regularly promotes and utilises a 'true' knowledge of subjects and indeed in a certain manner constitutes the very field of that truth. So, with Foucault, we view the 'subject' as a constructed entity, and this requires a methodological scepticism about both the ontological claims and ethical values which humanist systems of thought invest in the notion of subjectivity:

> Maybe the target nowadays is not to discover what we are, but to refuse what we are. We have to imagine and to build up what we could be to get rid of this kind of political 'double blind', which is the simultaneous individualization and totalization of modern power structures. The conclusion would be that the political, ethical, social, philosophical problem of our days is not to try and liberate the individual from the state and from the state's institutions, but to liberate us both from the state and from the type of individualization which is linked to the state. We have to promote new forms of subjectivity through the refusal of this kind of individuality which has been imposed upon us for several centuries.
>
> (Foucault 1982: 216)

Overall the concepts of social capital, and Foucault's work on power, can inform our understanding of social exclusion and connection by recognising inequalities and power differences within society, employing multi-dimensional mapping of spheres, settings, resources, communities, cultures and structures; and multi-directional dynamics of normative processes, trust, cohesion, access and identity.

The other side of exclusion – inclusion or connectedness?

Marmot (2004) summarises the considerable body of evidence that social standing directly affects health, and furthermore unpicks the (difficult) concept of 'social standing' into something far more concrete (and strongly related to social exclusion): 'Autonomy – how much control you have over your life – and the opportunities you have for full social engagement and participation are crucial for health, well-being and longevity' (Marmot 2004: 2). Putting this together with the discussions throughout this chapter on the complex inter-action of factors that create and recreate social exclusion, we can note a challenge in terms of building understanding as to how to formulate and implement policies that sidestep the twin dangers of: paying lip service to involvement and thereby fostering dependency through reinforcing lack of control and failing to tackle the issue of employment security and adequate recompense.

Given the importance of language in the operation of social exclusion, we therefore argue that the use of the term connectedness can more easily be seen to offer possibilities of agency and empowerment than the somewhat pater-nalistic notion of inclusion – inclusion is something done to people rather than by them.

A human rights approach to social exclusion

At a number of places already in this chapter we have alluded to the notion of rights in connection with the discussion of social exclusion. There are advantages to making these links much more explicit. Some writers con-ceptualise inclusion/exclusion in terms of various types of rights, for example Atkinson *et al.* (2002), discussing the EU, who utilise definitions based in terms of the ability to exercise, or not, basic social rights.

Room (1999) uses rights-based argumentation to describe social exclusion as the denial or non-realisation of civil, political and social rights of citizen-ship. Such a rights-based approach to the problem of social exclusion has much to recommend it, and has parallels to the rights-based approaches to health that have been increasingly developed since the 1990s (Gruskin *et al.* 2007; Beyrer *et al.* 2007; Singh *et al.* 2007). Renner *et al.* (2007) agree that a human rights-based approach should be the means to tackle social exclusion. Klasen (n.d.) suggests a rights-based approach to social exclusion has four advantages, similar to the advantages of Sen's capabilities-based approach (Sen 2000).

First, it emphasises that the inability to participate in, and be respected by, mainstream society is a violation of a basic right that should be open to all citizens (or residents). In contrast to a phrasing that positions social exclusion as a 'social' or 'welfare' issue, the rights-language considerably strengthens the case for society to ensure that it enables participation and integration of all its members; it also highlights the role of political, economic and social factors in creating (and maintaining) exclusion. Second, a rights-based approach does not demand uniformity of outcomes, but instead calls for equal freedoms for all – and it thus makes an important distinction between a choice of indivi-duals to not participate in mainstream society, and their inability to do so.

Third, it recognises the diversity of people in their ability to make use of opportunities. Thus calling for equal capabilities (or the ability to exercise civil and social citizenship rights) may necessitate extra efforts by society to provide equal capabilities to such people. An equal starting point (or 'equal opportunities') may not be enough to ensure equal capabilities. Finally, it focuses on ends and not on means. We return to the rights-based approach to social exclusion in Part 3 of the book.

Part 2

Insights into social exclusion and connectedness: theory, policy and practice

2.1 The other side of social exclusion: interrogating the role of the privileged in reproducing inequality[1]

Bob Pease

Introduction

As the chapters in this book demonstrate, social exclusion is a key concept used to understand various forms of inequality in contemporary capitalist societies. I argue in this chapter that while the concept of social exclusion has been important in illustrating the structural dimensions of unequal social relations and examining the costs of those relations for excluded groups, it has done little to address those of us who benefit most from existing social divisions and inequalities. Nor do most of the writings on social exclusion examine how these inequalities are reproduced by and through the daily practices and life-style pursuits of privileged groups.

In this chapter I will interrogate the concept of privilege as the other side of social exclusion and will argue that the lack of critical interrogation of the position of the privileged side of social divisions allows the privileged to reinforce their dominance. I aim to make privilege more visible and consider the extent to which those who are privileged can overcome their own self interest in the maintenance of dominance to enable them to challenge it.

Interrogating social exclusion and inclusion

Social exclusion has become a major concept in social policy research. Although it is often used to denote those marginalised by non-participation in the labour market, Lister (2000: 36) says that social exclusion 'is a multi-dimensional concept ... embracing a variety of ways in which people may be denied full participation in society'. It is clear, though, that the concept of social exclusion can be employed in very different ways depending on whether the primary objective is social cohesion or social justice (Lister 2000).

The opposite of social exclusion is seen to be 'social inclusion' which is defined as 'the attempt to re-integrate or increase the participation of marginalised groups within mainstream goals' (Barry 1998: 1). Sheppard (2006: 5) maintains that social exclusion and inclusion are 'two sides of the same coin'. Is social inclusion a solution to the issue of marginalisation or does it distract us from the need for fundamental social change?

Some writers distinguish between different interpretations of social exclusion. One version involves greater integration of excluded people into the dominant society (Sheppard 2006), while the other version focuses on the dominant group who are the sources of exclusion (Byrne 2005). However, what are the consequences of replacing discussions of equality with the concept of social inclusion? Edwards *et al.* (2001: 425) suggest that the notion of inclusion positions the excluded as deficient or deviant who need to conform to the prevailing norms. I am doubtful that the language of social inclusion can provide a basis for social change. As Anthias (2000: 839) has noted, 'subordination and economic exploitation can coexist under inclusion and in fact they constitute dis-empowering forms of inclusion'. Jones and Smythe (1999) suggest that the language of inclusion can actually perpetuate social exclusion.

Even in the more radical versions of social exclusion, the focus is almost always on the excluded. Somerville (2000) focuses on the opportunities and capacity of the excluded to resist the forces of exclusion. Byrne (1999) also emphasises the potential of the excluded to be organised through coalitions and social movements that are promoting social solidarity. More recently, however, Byrne (2005) has questioned whether social exclusion can be eliminated by interventions directed solely at the excluded.

Anthias (2000) identifies the tendency to identify persons as 'the excluded', and who are said to constitute varying degrees of exclusion from the normative ideals of the majority. In this regard, there is the danger that those seen as socially excluded may be portrayed as 'either passive victims or willing agents in their own denigration' (Anthias 2000: 838). The focus is thus on the process of producing 'a disqualified identity'. She maintains that the focus on the excluded 'focuses too much attention at the bottom of the scale and does not allow for looking at forms of inequality and hierarchy more generally' (Anthias 2000: 838). This shifts attention off the dominant group and reinforces the tendency of sociology to study 'downwards'.

Numerous writers have drawn attention to this focus on studying downwards. Bessant and Watts (1999: 309) for example, ask: 'Why don't we research the wealthy?' Jamrozik and Nocella (1998) similarly note that academics study 'the others' rather than studying 'ourselves'. They observe that 'There is multitude of studies of "deviance" of the poor, the disadvantaged, but relatively few systematically conducted studies of the affluent and of the powerful' (Jamrozik and Nocella 1998: 217).

Why is this so? Ferber (2003: 319) maintains quite simply that we 'have tended to ignore the issue of privilege because it implicates those in power'. This lack of a critical interrogation of privilege and internalised dominance allows dominant groups to reinforce their dominance. If we focus exclusively upon oppression and social exclusion, we reinforce the invisibility of privilege. The powerful and the privileged become invisible because they are subsumed under the 'normal and ordinary' (Byrne 2005: 57). Understanding the construction of privilege is necessary for a complete understanding of social exclusion.

Bailey (1998: 109) describes privilege as 'systematically conferred advantages individuals enjoy by virtue of their membership in dominant groups with access to resources and institutional power that are beyond the common advantages of marginalised citizens'. Sidanius and Pratto (1999) identify the main benefits that accrue from privilege: 'possession of a disproportionately large share of positive social value or all those material and symbolic things for which people strive. Examples of positive social value are such things as political authority and power, good and plentiful food, splendid homes, the best available health care, wealth and high social status' (Sidanius and Pratto 1999: 31–32). Individuals come to possess these benefits 'by virtue of his or her prescribed membership in a particular socially constructed group such as race, religion, clan, tribe, ethnic group or social class' (Sidanius and Pratto 1999: 32). An individual's privilege is thus more a product of their membership of privileged groups than it is of their individual capabilities.

To critically explore the concept of privilege, we need to identify the key characteristics. There are four main issues that I will discuss here: the invisibility of privilege by those who have it; the power of the privileged group to determine the social norm; the naturalisation of privilege and the sense of entitlement that accompanies privilege.

The invisibility of privilege

Most privilege is not recognised as such, by those who have it. In fact, 'one of the functions of privilege is to structure the world so that mechanisms of privileges are invisible – in the sense that they are unexamined – to those who benefit from them' (Bailey 1998: 112). Johnson (2001) observes how members of privileged groups either do not understand what others mean when they refer to them as privileged or they tend to get angry and defensive. Because privilege does not necessarily bring happiness and fulfilment, this will sometimes be used to deny the existence of privilege. These responses represent significant obstacles to the struggle for equality.

Members of privileged groups occupy what Rosenblum and Travis (1996) call an 'unmarked status'. By this they mean that people in unmarked categories do 'not require any special comment. Thus, the unmarked category tells us what a society takes for granted' (Rosenblum and Travis 1996: 142). One of the consequences of this is that members of privileged groups are unlikely to be aware of how others may not have access to the benefits that they receive and thus they are unlikely to be able to acknowledge the experiences of those who are marginalised. Many privileged individuals may thus oppress people without being aware of it. When people are unable to recognise their privilege because they are so focused on their oppression, they are unable to see their role in keeping others subordinated.

While members of dominant groups may intentionally oppress others, not all members of dominant groups behave in oppressive ways. However, the reproduction of oppression does not demand the intent of individuals. Ferree *et al.* (1999) discusses how, for example, white people gain privileges through 'the subordination ... of people of color, even if he or she is not personally exploiting or taking advantage of any person of color' (Ferree *et al.* 1999: 11).

The normativity of privilege

Privileged groups have become the model for 'normative human relations' and this explains in part why they do not want to know about the experiences of the excluded (Baker Miller 1995: 61). The privileged group comes to represent the hegemonic norm whereby 'white, thin male young heterosexual Christian and financially secure people come to embody what it means to be normal' (Perry 2001: 192). Perry (2001) observes that through the positioning of self and other, various dualisms are established in which forms of difference are devalued because they are seen as inferior, weak or subordinate in relation to the normal which is presented as superior, strong and dominant. The normativity of privilege means that this becomes the basis for measuring success and failure. Those who are not privileged are potentially regarded as aberrant and deviant. The establishment of this normative standard reproduces the negative valuation of difference. Because the privileged are regarded as 'normal', they are less likely to be studied or researched because the norm does not have to be 'marked'. Gender then, for example, becomes a code word for women and race becomes synonymous with people of colour.

The normativity of privilege provides some insight to the process of 'othering', as the flipside of the 'other' are the insiders who constitute the privileged group (Dominelli 2002). Pickering (2001: 73) reminds us 'that those who are "othered", are unequally positioned in relation to those who *do* the "othering"' (emphasis mine). The latter occupy a privileged space in which they define themselves in contrast to the others who are designated as different.

The naturalisation of privilege

The social divisions between the privileged and the oppressed are further reproduced through their attributed naturalness. Rather than seeing difference as being socially constructed, gender, race, sexuality and class are regarded as flowing from nature. Beliefs about social hierarchy as being natural provides a rationale for social dominance and absolves dominant groups from responsibility to address social inequalities (Gould 2000).

It is the belief in the 'God-given' or biological basis of dominance that reproduces social inequality. Members of privileged groups either believe that they have inherited the characteristics that give them advantages or they set out to consciously cover up the socially constructed basis of their dominance (Wonders 2000). When we understand the way in which difference is socially constructed, we are more able to develop strategies for challenging inequality.

Part of the process of interrogating dominant identities is to question their appearance of naturalness. As Tillner reports (1997: 3): 'It means to lay open their contingency, their dependency on power relations and to particularise them'. He proposes an important strategy of endeavouring to represent non-dominant identities as 'normal' and representing dominant identities as 'particular' as a way of subverting the tendency for dominant groups to always represent themselves as 'the universal'.

The sense of entitlement associated with privilege

Another aspect of privilege is the sense of entitlement that members of privileged groups feel about their status. As Rosenblum and Travis (1996: 141) state: 'The sense of entitlement that one has a right to be respected, acknowledged, protected and rewarded – is so much taken for granted by those of us in non-stigmatised statuses, that they are often shocked and angered when it is denied them'. Lyn (1992), in reflecting upon her own situation as a white woman, describes how she had come to believe that she deserved whatever benefits and status she had attained because she had struggled for them. She did not recognise how her class and race facilitated that struggle.

Many writers have connected men's sense of male entitlement to violence against women. As Connell (2000: 3) puts it: 'From a long history of gender relations, many men have a sense of entitlement to respect, deference, and service from women. If women fail to give it, some men will see this as bad conduct which ought to be punished'. She also notes that some men will regard women's challenge to male entitlement as a threat to their masculinity.

We thus need to understand more clearly how privileged group members' sense of entitlement is subjectively experienced and socially constructed. Hatty (2000: 58) has noted, for example, that 'men may employ particular rhetorical devices to reinforce the contours of their version of reality of their entitlement to use violence'. Adams et al. (1995) identify the ways in which men use language to reinforce their assumptions about male dominance. Men construct what Adams et al. (1995) call a 'discourse of natural entitlement' which enables them to believe that they are designed to dominate women. These discourses legitimate men's use of violence against women.

Towards an intersectional theory of privilege

While different forms of exclusion are distinct, they are also interrelated and mutually reinforcing. This approach means that people who are excluded may also participate in the exclusion of others. It is necessary then for people who are excluded to not only struggle against their own exclusion but also to confront their own privilege and internalised dominance. I recognise, however, that the onus to change should be greater for those who have access to multiple levels of privilege. In advocating a greater level of responsibility by members of dominant groups for the maintenance of privilege, I also acknowledge that an understanding of privilege necessitates a structural analysis that identifies the systemic nature of privilege.

What an intersectional analysis makes clear is that 'all groups possess varying degrees of penalty and privilege in one historically created system' (Collins 1991: 225). While people find it relatively easy to identify their experience of oppression and exclusion, they often find it harder to recognise how their thoughts and actions uphold the subordination of others. Some people may struggle against their oppression but at the same time maintain their access to various dimensions of privilege. When people are able to define themselves in terms of one or more forms of oppression, they may not feel the need to acknowledge themselves as benefiting from another form or forms of oppression (Wildman and Davis 2000). Given that most people can be seen to exhibit both some degree of penalty and privilege, it is equally important for individuals to see themselves as belonging to dominant groups as well as to excluded groups.

As those groups who are both excluded and privileged start to examine their privilege, we need to be careful that these groups are not asked to take more than their share of the responsibility for the reproduction of privilege. Razack (1998) observes, for example, that white women's writing is judged more harshly than white men's writing. However, following Razack (1998), I think that groups who are oppressed or excluded on one dimension need to acknowledge their complicity with other relations of domination and subordination. We all need to locate ourselves in the social relations of domination and oppression. If everyone were simply privileged or just subordinated then the analysis of systems of privilege would be easier.

The internalisation of dominance and privilege

A concept that has been used to understand some of the ways in which privileged people sustain their dominant position is 'internalised domination'. Pheterson (1986: 147) defines internalised domination as 'the incorporation and acceptance by individuals within a dominant group of prejudices against others'. The concept of internalised domination may explain in part 'why significant numbers of people from the dominant group seem to hold oppressive thoughts and exert oppressive behaviour but do not consider themselves to be oppressive' (Mullaly 2002: 145).

Tillner (1997: 2) usefully takes this notion of internalised domination a little further by defining dominance 'as a form of identity practice that constructs a difference which legitimises dominance and grants the agent of dominance the illusion of a superior identity'. In this process, the identities of others are invalidated. Thus, because dominance is socially constructed and psychically internalised, to challenge it, we will need to explore different models of identity and construct subjectivities that are not based on domination and subordination.

It is not possible for members of dominant groups to escape completely the internalisation of dominance (Johnson 2001). Negative ideas and images are deeply embedded in the culture and it is unlikely that men, whites and heterosexuals will not be affected by sexism, racism and homophobia. As noted earlier, prejudice is not necessarily always consciously enacted by members of dominant groups.

Bourdieu's work is useful in explaining how various forms of inequality are reproduced and internalised. He formulated the term 'habitus' to explain how 'a system of stable dispositions' lead people to see the world from a particular perspective (Bourdieu 1977a). Unlike Marxist and radical humanist views, however, which outline how people's ideas and consciousness are shaped by dominant ideologies, Bourdieu emphasises how dominant ideologies are incorporated into the body. He argues that dispositions are 'beyond the grip of conscious control and therefore not amenable to transformations or corrections' (Bourdieu 2001: 95). Bourdieu regards a person's habitus as 'a direct product of the person's structural situation; it is the psychological embodiment of the objective conditions in which one lives' (Hurst 2001: 198).

The concepts of internalised domination and habitus help us to understand the seeming paradox that Minow (1990) identifies in relation to those who publicly criticise social inequality, while at the same time engaging in practices that perpetuate these inequalities. While she emphasises the task of examining and reformulating our assumptions about the social world, she acknowledges that this requires more than individuals learning to think differently, because of the ways in which the individual's thinking is shaped by institutional and cultural forces. Thus, while it is important for individuals to acknowledge the privileges they have and to speak out against them, it is impossible to simply relinquish privilege as an act of will.

Given the complexity of the issues facing members of privileged groups, how are they to respond when they are challenged about their privilege? How do egalitarian individuals live their lives in ways that are congruent with their values and beliefs? It is easy to feel despair when one is constantly challenged by subordinate groups. Are there any ways of resolving these dilemmas?

Privilege and positionality

Those in dominant groups will be more likely than those in subordinate groups to argue that existing inequalities are legitimate or natural. Sidanius and Pratto (1999: 61) formulate the notion of 'social dominance orientation' to explain 'the value that people place on non-egalitarianism and hierarchically-structured relations among people and social groups'. They argue that people develop an 'orientation towards social dominance' by virtue of the power and status of their primary group. This social dominance orientation is largely a product of one's membership within dominant groups, although they seem to allow that some members of dominant groups may identify with subordinates.

Most members of privileged groups appear to actively defend privileged positions. In this context, government interventions aimed at addressing inequality and mobilisation by socially excluded groups (important as they both are) seem unlikely to fundamentally change the social relations of dominance and subordination (Crowfoot and Chesler 2003). What likelihood is there then that members of privileged groups might form alliances with excluded groups? What would encourage them to do so?

Just as oppressed groups have a range of strategies available to them to respond to their oppression, Dominelli (2002) identifies three strategies that dominant groups can utilise to respond to concerns or questions about their privilege: demarcationalist, incorporationist and egalitarian. Demarcationalists view the world through a hierarchical lens and endeavour to hold on to and increase their power and resources to maintain their privileged position. Incorporationalists may support incremental changes but they also want to retain existing social divisions. Egalitarians reject the social order that grants them privileges because they recognise the injustice associated with their position.

Harding (1995) believes that it is possible for members of dominant groups to develop the capacity to see themselves from the perspective of those in subordinated groups. Because subjectivity is generated through social processes, she argues that dominant subjectivities can also be changed by these processes. Dominant groups do not necessarily form a homogeneous network of shared interests, making it possible for members of dominant groups to 'resist the usual assumptions and orientations of those groups' (Sawhney 1995: 284). This is consistent with my experience of constructing a profeminist men's standpoint in researching the experiences of men (Pease 2000).

Bailey's (2000) argument that members of dominant groups can develop what she calls 'traitorous identities', adds support to this position. She differentiates between those who are unaware of their privilege and those who are critically cognisant of their privilege. Traitors are thus those who refuse to reproduce their privilege and who challenge the worldviews that dominant groups are expected to adhere to. These dominant group members are able to identify with the experiences of oppressed groups. It is from this basis that white people will challenge racism and that men will challenge patriarchy. So while it is difficult for members of privileged groups to critically appraise their own position, it is not impossible.

The process of developing a traitorous identity involves learning to see the world through the experiences of the oppressed (Bailey 2000). This may not be fully possible but members of dominant groups can make a choice about accepting or rejecting their part in the establishment. Members of privileged groups have a responsibility to deconstruct their own discourse. As Johnson (2001: 166) says, it is more important for 'members of privileged groups to work with others on issues of privilege rather than trying to help members of subordinate groups'.

Privilege as structured action: doing dominance

It is through the processes of accomplishing gender, race and class, etcetera, that social dominance is reproduced. Rather than seeing concepts like race, gender and class as reified categories, we should be more interested in the processes of gendering, racialising and classing. In this project, I draw upon the work of Fenstermaker and West (2002a) who set out to analyse how race, gender and class constitute 'ongoing methodical and situated accomplishments' (2002a: 75). They analyse how people conduct themselves in specific situations to understand 'how the most fundamental divisions of our society are legitimated and maintained' (Fenstermaker and West 2002a: 78).

Messerschmidt (1997: 4) similarly, in discussing crime as 'structured action', emphasises how 'the social construction of gender, race and class involves a situated, social and interactional accomplishment'. Gender, race and class are thus a series of activities that we do in specific situations that are influenced by structural constraints. Because they involve accomplishments enacted by human agents, it is possible to resist the reproduction of social structures. Talking specifically about men, for example, Messerschmidt (1993) argues that masculinity is something that has to be accomplished in specific social contexts. It is 'what men do under specific constraints and varying degrees of power' (Messerschmidt 1993: 81).

When we act in the world, we are not just operating within structural constraints. Rather, we are also determining the nature of those structures through our actions and interactions. The structures which oppress us then are not only contextual. They are also constituted through our actions. This means that we can challenge those arrangements by engaging in 'inappropriate' racial or gender behaviour.

Various commentators have argued that this approach neglects the structural dimensions of inequality. Maldonado (2002: 85) for example, says that there is insufficient acknowledgement of 'the constraints imposed by the macro-level forces in the social environment'. O'Brien and Howard (1998: xiv) also argue that this approach 'obscures institutional and structural power relations'. Weber (2002: 89) says that Fenstermaker and West obscure 'the mechanisms of power in the production and maintenance of racism, class and sexism' because therein 'exclusive attention to face to face interaction, macro social structural processes such as institutional arrangements are rendered invisible'. In Weber's view, the structural dimensions of social inequalities cannot be transformed by 'the attitudes and actions of a few actors in everyday interactions' (2002: 90).

Certainly, we must acknowledge the importance of locating class, gender and race relations in the context of institutional structures. We must also accept that 'gender, and race, class and compulsory heterosexuality extend deep into the unconscious and outward into social structure and material interests' (Thorne 2002: 85). However, how useful is it to establish a duality of micro and macro forces? Why must structure and action be represented as an either/or opposition? Because I am interested in opposition, resistance and change, social action that challenges the processes of 'differentiating persons according to sex categories, race categories and/or class categories ... undermines the legitimacy of existing institutional arrangements' (Fenstermaker and West 2002b: 99).

O'Brien (1998: 25) captures the complexity well when she says that 'we are socially constituted subjects who navigate webs of opportunities and obstacles not necessarily of our own choosing'. Furthermore, I agree wholeheartedly with Collins *et al.* (2002: 81) who argue that the concept of interlocking oppressions must involve a recognition of both 'macro-level connections' at the level of social structures and 'micro-level processes' which describes how individuals experience their positions within the hierarchies of domination and oppression. In challenging the dichotomisation of micro and macro forces, we must view the relationship between social structure and social action as 'dynamic and reciprocal' (Messerschmidt 1997: 14). While social structure is reproduced by the widespread and continual actions of individuals, it also 'produces subjects'. Individuals do not simply produce gender, race and class in a vacuum. Rather, they are reproduced and constrained by institutional settings such as families, workplaces and the state.

We must move beyond this conflict between 'social constructionist' and 'structuralist' approaches. We must interrogate privilege at interactional, cultural and structural levels at the same time that we explore the intersections of privilege with social exclusion.

Conclusion

In this chapter I have argued that to gain a broader understanding of the processes that produce social exclusion, we need to focus on the individuals and groups who benefit from those processes and activities. We must all recognise how we are enmeshed in the social relations of dominance and subordination that we criticise and that we too are likely to have internalised dominance in varying degrees (Brewer 1997).

Although I teach courses about and write articles and books on dominant forms of masculinity and privilege, I still benefit from gender, race, class and sexual privilege. In what ways does the academic discourse exclude the voices of marginalised people? Is it enough for us to be simply critical of our positioning, while doing nothing to change the material conditions that produce it? Obviously not, but if we own our positionality, we at least challenge the view that the white middle-class male perspective represents some form of transcendent truth. To challenge this ethos, more white middle-class men will need to read and reflect upon the writings by those who are marginalised and excluded. We need to feel distressed by these experiences and come to disapprove of our unearned advantages which are conferred upon us simply because of our membership of privileged groups. Such distress may be the starting point for more of us to challenge the systems that benefit us unfairly.

Notes

1 An earlier, shorter version of the discussion of the characteristics of privilege was published as part of the following article: Pease. B. (2006) 'Encouraging critical reflections on privilege in Social Work', *Practice Reflexions*, Vol. 1, No. 1, pp. 15–25.

2.2 Professional discretion and social exclusion

Beth R. Crisp

Introduction

In 1770 Samuel Johnson, who developed the English dictionary, observed that 'a decent provision for the poor is the true test of civilization ... The condition of the lower orders, the poor especially, was the true mark of national discrimination' (in Harris 2000: 61). Slightly later in 1776, the Scottish economist Adam Smith claimed:

> no society can surely be flourishing and happy, of which the far greater part of the members are poor and miserable. It is but equity, besides, that they who feed, clothe and lodge the whole body of the people, should have such a share of the produce of their own labour as to be themselves tolerably well fed, clothed and lodged.
>
> (in Harris 2000: 62)

More than two hundred years after these pronouncements, I found myself as a first year social work student assigned to a 14-week placement in a welfare agency located in one of the poorest and most stigmatised suburbs of Melbourne. Furthermore, the families we worked with were among the most disadvantaged and excluded within this community. While they had many issues, a lot of energy went into responding to immediate crises in respect of basic needs in food, clothing and housing. Every three months the agency received a small fund of money which could be distributed to service users who needed 'emergency relief'. Compared to the needs we encountered everyday, this money was nothing more than a token, and was always expended well before the next instalment would arrive. Decisions needed to be made as to how this money would be distributed and as a member of the social work team, I found myself making recommendations to the agency manager about this. I soon learnt that that this required the exercise of professional discretion as there were no formalised rules about how much could be provided in particular situations as indeed every situation was different.

Two decades later, I am a social work educator, and a key component of my teaching involves exploring dimensions of social exclusion on the basis that 'social work ... is ... almost exclusively concerned with the most dependent and least economically successful minority groups in the populations' (Pinker 1989: 85). In the program in which I teach, we have a stated commitment to the principles of anti-oppressive practice. We hope that our students will learn to appreciate that some approaches to practice have the potential to redress experiences of social exclusion while other approaches may reinforce exclusion. At the same time, students have to learn that despite how deserving they may warrant a situation, their ability to respond will be constrained by a range of factors beyond their control:

> Social work ... agencies are given specific responsibilities and powers through statute, and social workers ... have to practice within legislative frameworks and organisational policies and procedures. They have to balance the needs, rights, responsibilities and resources of people with those of the wider community, and provide appropriate levels of support, advocacy, care, protection and control.
>
> (Central Council for Education and Training in Social Work 1995: 16)

Balancing the needs and rights of numerous and diverse stakeholders in an environment of limited resources, and exercising professional discretion, also describes my work as an educator. This is particularly so whenever I am selecting new students into the social work degree or making determinations about current students.

The professional gatekeeper

Notwithstanding the key aim of social work education being to prepare students for professional practice, course providers have often been viewed as 'gatekeepers' whose task it is to screen out those unsuitable for professional practice (Moore and Unwin 1991). This typically commences at the point of seeking entry into a course of study. It would seem that while often quick to embrace the opportunities to promote social inclusion, social work educators frequently find themselves policing entry and maintaining the exclusiveness of the profession. While such actions are invariably done with the best possible motives, we risk further marginalisation of some already excluded populations (Crisp and Gillingham 2008).

Since its establishment in 1977, Deakin University has placed a high priority on offering educational opportunities to potential students who demonstrate aptitude for university study but due to various reasons require a flexible mode of delivery in order to access higher education. Hence, many of the university's courses, including social work, are offered so that students can study either full or part-time and in on or off campus modes. Students who successfully complete the final year of secondary school in Australia obtain an ENTER score which is a national ranking of achievement used by universities to select applicants into undergraduate courses. However, applicants for the

Bachelor of Social Work often apply for entry under Deakin University's Access and Equity Program. The program aims to offer a substantial minority of places to applicants who have experienced educational disadvantage which either did not allow them to complete their schooling, or if they did complete their schooling, to achieve an ENTER score which reflects their ability to succeed at further study. Categories of disadvantage include socioeconomic disadvantage, having a disability or other health impairment, or living in a rural or remote area. Such applicants need to demonstrate the capacity to succeed at university studies but can do this by alternative means such as by having completed courses since leaving school, or through relevant paid or voluntary work experience. Many of these applicants will have extensive experience in the welfare sector as workers and/or as service users. Furthermore, some will have completed vocational qualifications equivalent or higher than final year secondary studies but do not have an ENTER score which enables them to be ranked directly against successful secondary school completers. Also, a substantial number of applicants for our undergraduate social work degree have already undertaken previous studies in higher education, sometimes demonstrating much greater aptitude for university study than an ENTER score obtained some years earlier might have predicted.

As occurs in many Australian universities, Deakin University selects social work students on the basis of their written applications and supporting documentation including academic transcripts, details of previous employment, personal statements and applications for special consideration. On the basis of all this information, selection officers have to determine which applicants are best able to succeed in their studies. Conversely, I also had to identify any applicants who should not be offered a place on the grounds that they have not been able to demonstrate academic capacity to complete the four year social work degree program. While the university provides some guidance to assist selection officers to identify those applicants to whom an offer of a place should be made, the process necessarily relies on selection officers being able to exercise a degree of professional discretion in the form of academic judgements.

Importantly, the use of professional discretion during student selection allows for the possibility of selecting some students who, as a result of social exclusionary processes, have been denied an opportunity to succeed in the final year of secondary schooling. As at May 2007, 28.7 per cent of Australian adults aged 20 to 64 had not completed a final year of secondary schooling or completed any post-school qualification. A further 18.4 per cent had completed certificate level qualifications only since leaving school which may have been undertaken without completing a final secondary year at school (ABS 2007a). Many applicants to Deakin University's social work degree are in these categories, but bring a wealth of experience to their studies and have proved excellent students despite not having formally completed their secondary schooling.

A second category of access and equity applications comes from applicants who have completed their final year of secondary schooling but suffered some degree of disadvantage during their schooling which left them unable to fulfil their potential and gain an ENTER score which is a realistic appraisal of their abilities. Requests for special consideration range from those who out-line situations which appear trivial and not outside the norm, to requests from students who have completed their schooling in what can only be described as incredibly adverse circumstances and evoke a response of sheer admiration for having done as well as they have done. Again it becomes a question of academic judgement as to whether an applicant has a better chance of succeeding in the course than would be suggested by their ENTER score alone.

In making academic judgements as to who should be selected into a finite number of places in a social work degree, it is assumed that the selection officer has the expertise to exercise professional discretion appropriately. At Deakin University, this has required me to make judgements about an indi-vidual's academic capacity to undertake a course of university study. The principles of student selection in higher education require Australian uni-versities to take into account equal opportunities legislation, which imposes a duty on them not to discriminate against students according to age, gender, race, disability, sexual orientation or criminal background (Shardlow 2000). This differs from the role of selection officers in some overseas social work courses who are more explicitly charged with making moral judgements as to who is fit and proper to be a social worker, and consequently who is suitable to undertake a course of study leading to qualification as a social worker (Crisp 2006). This has substantial implications when considering applicants who have substantial criminal records.

Applicants with criminal records

Occasionally in the process of selecting students, an applicant discloses that he or she has a criminal record, or even that they are currently serving a prison sentence. This in itself is not grounds to exclude an applicant for study at Deakin University, but does raise a series of questions around the junction between promoting social inclusion, my professional duty of care, and how professional discretion is administered in this situation.

It has been argued that imprisonment is the ultimate form of social exclu-sion (Smith and Stewart 1998). Moreover, persons who are at greatest risk of experiencing social exclusion as a result of factors such as poverty, lack of education, unemployment and/or being a member of a racial minority, are disproportionately likely to have become prisoners (Mair and May 1997; Smith and Stewart 1998). In Australia, this is particularly an issue for indi-genous Australians (Wilson 1997). So extensive and enduring is their exclu-sion, that many offenders accept it as a 'fact of life' (Smith and Stewart 1998). Consequently, it has been proposed that promoting social inclusion is essen-tial, not only for reintegrating former prisoners into society, but to reduce the likelihood of re-offending (Clements 2004; Smith and Stewart 1998).

One of the most common methods of promoting social inclusion among prisoners is through the provision of education and training. Research indicates that those who undertake studies while imprisoned are not only more employable and have significantly higher incomes than those who were not involved in a prison education program (Fabelo 2002), but also lower rates of re-offending in the first few years post-release (Chappell 2004). While the research literature has very much focused on the potential of education to reduce economic exclusion, one might readily surmise that the unstated aim of some prison education programs is to enhance social connectedness by increasing employability. A more cynical view (and not one I would espouse) might be that education enables an individual to move away from the criminal sub-culture in which they are supposedly enmeshed, to moving with a so-called 'better' class of individuals.

Notwithstanding the fact that offenders who have undertaken post-school studies are more likely to gain employment than those with less formal education (Holzer *et al.* 2003), the extent to which graduate offenders obtain employment in their field of qualification is unclear in previous research. It may be that graduates with a criminal record are being employed in positions requiring less skill than those for which they are qualified. To some extent, employability in particular professions may be determined by the type of offence committed and employer's perceptions as to its relevance to the position applied for (Albright and Denq 1996). Graduate positions generally involve significant levels of trust (Waldfogel 1994), but a criminal record can be perceived by employers as suggesting a lack of trustworthiness (Holzer *et al.* 2003), a position which may be reflected in corporate policies pertaining to the recruitment and retention of staff (Taxman *et al.* 2002). But even if these are not explicit policy, employer beliefs certainly contribute to an offender's likelihood of obtaining employment (Fletcher 2001). Furthermore, there may be legal barriers preventing persons with a criminal record from obtaining or retaining employment in many professions (Heinrich 2000). Professional registration, where it exists, typically requires applicants to demonstrate 'good moral character' which can be perceived by those controlling access to employment as an insurmountable problem for persons with a criminal record (Heinrich 2000).

Over the past two decades, several writers from both the United Kingdom and the United States have debated the risks associated with employing social workers who have criminal records and consequently, the appropriateness of allowing persons who have a criminal record to participate in a program of education leading to qualification as a social worker (for an overview of this literature see Crisp and Gillingham 2008). While some have argued that admission of persons with a criminal conviction should occur on a case by case basis (Perry 2004; Scott and Zeiger 2000), others have argued vehemently against this (Magen and Emerman 2000). Difficulties in ensuring placements on courses, and subsequent jobs on graduation, can be secured for students with criminal convictions has sometimes been used to justify screening of offenders at the point of selection into a degree program in social welfare (Perry 2004). However, this may lead to presumptions as to local welfare agencies having the presence of policies, e.g. forbidding employment of convicted offenders, which in fact may not exist (Miller and Rodwell 1997; Smith 1999).

Rather than taking the line of some other universities and automatically rejecting applicants to social work degrees who disclose any serious criminal convictions, the approach at Deakin University has been for such applicants to be considered on precisely the same grounds as any other applicant, namely whether they have the academic ability to undertake and succeed at a course of studies. Information for prospective applicants does however warn that in order to complete the placement requirements of the Bachelor of Social Work degree, students will be required to obtain a Police Records Check prior to each placement, and may also need to obtain a Working with Children Check. This generates the occasional query from applicants who can then be provided with advice as to the likelihood of the university being able to obtain the necessary placements for them to complete the degree. Potential applicants can then make an informed decision as to whether to apply for a place in the social work degree.

Professional discretion

The use of professional discretion, as I have described above, has enabled me to select some students into a degree program at university on the basis of a much wider, and often highly individualised set of criteria than simply considering the ENTER scores obtained by successful school finishers. This has in the past enabled the university to contribute to overcoming experiences of social exclusion, particularly in respect of individuals whose exclusion has impacted on their educational attainment. For such individuals, obtaining a university qualification in a field in which there are numerous job opportunities is likely to have long-term benefits for the individuals involved and for some has the potential to break cycles of intergenerational poverty. This includes individuals who did not have the opportunity to complete their schooling, who live in rural areas where educational opportunities are limited, who have been victims of violence or family breakdown, have a serious illness or disability, grown up in a family which was impoverished and/or experienced other difficult circumstances. The university also has programs which aim to provide higher education opportunities to indigenous Australians.

Although it is often suggested that the ability to exercise discretion is what distinguished a professional from a functionary (Baker 2005; Clark 2005), the exercise of professional discretion necessarily involves a degree of subjectivity and the potential for different outcomes depending on who is actually making the decisions, even when using the same general principles:

> The beliefs held by citizens about society's responsibility for the dis-
> advantaged and vulnerable among them and about how assistance ...

should be designed form the moral conditions for discretion. On a general level, most people can agree on fundamental principles of action. Reaching consensus on how those principles should be concretised in specific cases is, however, a trickier matter and one that causes difficulties for street-level bureaucrats.

(Dunér and Nordström 2006: 430)

A study involving 52 frontline workers whose role it was to assess access to benefits under California's Welfare to Work program, CalWORKS, were asked to determine which of a range of benefits should be provided to a fictitious client and her family. Participants in this study were also asked to comment on the extent to which each of a list of 24 factors or issues concerning the client and her family influenced their decision making. Finally, participants were asked what, if any, information about this client suggested that the goal of finding work for her would be problematic. Overall there was a lack of consensus on almost every factor as to whether it should be used to form an assessment and how it would influence an assessment. Not surprisingly, participants identified a diverse range of short and long term goals for the client within the limits allowed by the program (Johnson *et al.* 2006).

Like the CalWORKS assessors, my role in selecting students places me as what Robert Lipsky (1980) has described as a 'street-level bureaucrat'. Lipsky applies this definition to a wide range of professionals who work at the interface between the organisations which employ them and the public, and whose work involves them interpreting policy imperatives when faced with individuals in diverse circumstances. As such;

The work of street-level bureaucrats is multifaceted and of a contradictory nature. Demands and expectations are imposed on them from a variety of sources ... Their tasks entail making decisions based on the needs of the individual within the confines of prevailing policy. They are forced to make necessary prioritisations when they must bring into alignment public objectives and the individual's need for assistance and support with available resources.

(Dunér and Nordström 2006: 426)

There are some particular dilemmas arising from my role as a selection officer which I share with a relatively small pool of colleagues in universities who have a similar role, and most readers might not relate to these. However, the question as to how use of discretion can promote or hinder social inclusion is potentially an issue for a very wide range of professionals, both within and beyond the human services and higher education sectors.

The existence of discretionary provision arrangements typically makes assumptions that the decision makers will be appropriately qualified to perform their duties (Stein-Roggenbuck 2005). The effectiveness of discretionary measures in reducing social exclusion does however require that professionals are aware of discretionary measures open to them and being willing to adopt a discretionary approach when required (Palley 2004). Nevertheless, in situations in which decision making appears highly routinised, there will often be some workers who seem to be able to find ways to introduce a degree of discretion which recognises and addresses various forms of disadvantage or exclusion (Baker 2005; Evans and Harris 2004). This no doubt reflects the fact that for many professionals, being required to make decisions but having no discretion leads to alienation from the work (Cyrus and Vogel 2003).

While I have outlined a case as to why professional discretion has its place in professional practice, it nevertheless retains the ability to be problematic. Those at greatest risk of social exclusion may in fact benefit least from discretionary provisions (Stein-Roggenbuck 2005; Triandafyllidou 2003). Knowing what information to provide, and in what format this might influence a decision is essential (Lipsky 1980), but those who are most excluded may be further disadvantaged in such circumstances. Professional discretion is a potentially powerful tool in addressing social exclusion, but only if used appropriately (Evans and Harris 2004).

2.3 Not measuring up: low-income women receiving welfare benefits

Kay Cook

Introduction

The central notion of this chapter is that every person has the right to an elemental standard of social life, as a citizenship entitlement. However, segments of our society, such as women who rely on government payments as their primary source of income, do not enjoy full social citizenship entitlements and are instead socially excluded. Using data from in-depth qualitative interviews, I outline participants' experiences of stigma, marginalisation and exclusion. I posit that these experiences are the result of policy failure as financial assistance policies fail to fully provide these women with their social citizenship entitlements.

Social citizenship and the provision of welfare

Social citizenship, first introduced by T.H. Marshall (1950) as a subset of general citizenship, 'exists when a nation's laws and social provisions override de facto disadvantage based on ascriptive difference and personal misfortune' (Higgins and Ramina 2000: 137). The crux of Marshall's theory is that social citizenship is designed to lessen the differentiating effects of the market and enable citizens to participate in society to their fullest. The most common benefits associated with social citizenship are welfare benefits, as the welfare system plays an enormous role in administering entitlements to financially marginalised citizens. Such economic transfers are designed to lessen the differentiating effects of the market to enable those both employed and unemployed 'to share to the full in the social heritage and to live the life of a civilized being according to the standards prevailing in society' (Marshall 1950: 11).

The right to full participation in society is theoretically and unconditionally accorded equally to all citizens; however, this is problematic for low-income women as requirements for single parents' welfare receipt are conditional on attachment to the workforce. In Australia in 2005 the welfare benefit system was reformed to move single parents from welfare to work (Commonwealth of Australia 2005). These reforms, enacted in 2005 but discursively promoted in policy since the early 2000s, have shifted the focus of welfare away from issues of social citizenship and onto issues of economic individualism (Cook and Marjoribanks 2005). In this climate of personal responsibility, economic rationalism and reducing welfare expenditure, welfare policies mediate marginalised citizens' opportunities for social participation and shape the stigma experienced by recipients.

The social exclusion of welfare recipients

Social exclusion is a concept 'related to notions of poverty, hardship, deprivation and marginalisation' (Peace 2001: 17), which can be defined as 'disintegration from common cultural processes, lack of participation in social activities, alienation from decision-making and civic participation, and barriers to employment and material resources' (Reid 2004: 27). Examining welfare benefits as a mediator of social exclusion has gained political acceptability primarily in the United Kingdom where welfare policies specifically aim to lead people out of social exclusion through participation in paid work (Levitas 1998). Levitas's analysis of these policies revealed three discourses of social exclusion focusing on financial redistribution, social integration through paid work, or the moral fortitude of welfare recipients. These discourses are also evident in Australia where welfare policies focus simultaneously on promoting paid work and monitoring the moral behaviour of recipients (see for example Cook and Marjoribanks 2005; Carney 2007). This has implications for recipients' sense of exclusion and social citizenship, as pejorative policies can undermine the 'inclusive' aims they set out to achieve. For example, on 1 July 2006 the Australian federal government enacted the *Employment and workplace relations legislation amendment (Welfare to work and other measures) Act 2005 (No. 154)* which aims to move single parents from welfare to work.

The Australian government describes the benefits of employment for people receiving welfare benefits as 'higher incomes', 'better participation in mainstream economic life' (Costello 2005: 3), and improvements to 'wellbeing' (Commonwealth of Australia 2005: 132). However, these benefits are yet to be demonstrated and overseas experiences of welfare-to-work programs show mixed results. For example, qualitative studies of single mothers' experiences of moving from welfare to work have documented low wages, few job advancement opportunities, and continued reliance on welfare benefits and family for additional financial and in-kind support, such as health insurance and childcare (Litt *et al.* 2000; Dean and Coulter 2006). Further, while on average single parents in paid work have higher incomes than those reliant on income support, overseas research suggests that labour market participation by single parents does not necessarily ameliorate poverty (Baker and Tippin 2002; Walter 2002; Williamson and Salkie 2005). However, Centrelink (2005: 2), the Australian government agency responsible for the delivery of welfare services, asserts that 'paid work provides not only the money to live on and raise a family, but also improves self-esteem and provides a connection to the community'. Research suggests, however, that for both single mothers returning to work from welfare and for those who remain on benefits, the outcomes are often less optimistic (Baker and Tippin 2002; Hildebrandt and Kelber 2005).

In this chapter, I seek to describe the experience of low-income women receiving welfare benefits in Australia to explore how welfare receipt shapes their social exclusion. In order to explore low-income women's experience of social exclusion and welfare receipt, interviews were conducted with 28 women in receipt of welfare benefits.

Women receiving welfare benefits

Of the women interviewed, seven were married or in de facto relationships, 15 were separated, widowed or divorced, and six were single. With regards to family type, 18 women had at least one child under the age of 16, three women had adult children, and seven women had no children. One woman lived in a share-house environment, whereas all of the others lived either alone or with their immediate family, including children and partners if applicable.

While all of the women interviewed received some type of government benefit, six also worked part-time, three were students and 19 were neither employed nor undertaking further study. This group of 19 women included 12 home-makers and stay-at-home mothers, two women classified as 'jobseekers', two women with disabilities, one woman receiving an aged-pension, and two who were in receipt of sickness or injury benefits. Sixteen of the 28 women were under the age of 40.

The following description of the women's experiences begins from the analysis of two statements made by participants, which encapsulated their experience of social exclusion and social citizenship. These statements were:

> The more you stay at home the less self-esteem you have. You become a hermit really. I've got the stage where I don't want to leave the house anymore.
>
> (Christine[1])

> So when I'm stuck at home by myself I feel more confident because it's more like I'm in my fantasy world where I am in control and everything's perfect and no one's judging me.
>
> (Irene)

These statements have direct relevance to issues of social citizenship and social exclusion as these experiences are not indicative of sharing in the social heritage or living to the standards prevailing in society. Unravelling these statements to identify the basis of such exclusion is the grounds for the following analysis. The purpose of providing the findings as an unfolding analysis is to enable the reader to take the same analytical journey as myself. By documenting key analysis decisions and directions, the reader can judge for themselves the perspective taken by the researcher and to what extent it is useful for their own work. This is similar to the style of Becker (1993) in his process-oriented article 'How I learned what a crock was' where results are presented as an unfolding story where each layer of meaning, influence and understanding is revealed, and is reflected upon in light of the knowledge gained previously.

To summarise the two accounts, Christine states that she has less self-esteem as a result of staying at home, whereas Irene contends that she is more confident. The point of this exercise is not to determine which of these statements is 'true', but, rather, under what social circumstances the two statements can be compatible. As this process unfolds, the following analysis will draw upon not only the experiences of Christine and Irene, but all of the participants to provide a detailed account of how they experienced social citizenship and social exclusion.

Unravelling low-income women's social exclusion

The following analysis begins from the previous two statements which identify self-esteem as an issue for low-income women receiving welfare benefits, and a key to understanding their marginalisation and social exclusion. Healey (2002: 1) defines self-esteem as 'a sense of personal efficacy and a sense of personal worth. It is the integrated sum of self-confidence and self-respect. It is the conviction that one is competent to live and worthy of living'. Christine speaks of her self-esteem being eroded by being at home and presumably isolated (as a 'hermit') whereas Irene talks about being more confident when she is not being judged. The overall result, however, is that these women are socially excluded as they remain at home due to issues related to self-esteem.

The first question to be asked of the data, therefore, is 'why is it that one woman experiences increased self-esteem and another experiences decreased self-esteem as a result of the same situation'? In both cases the women are not receiving feedback from others. For Christine this reduces her self-esteem whereas for Irene this increases her self-confidence. It is feasible, therefore, that the type of feedback received or not received is important. Christine lacks positive feedback now that she is at home, whereas Irene feels better because she lacks negative feedback. These assumptions, however, are by no means taken as given. What is now required is a thorough examination of this issue, to be tested and refined through the following data analysis, in order to develop an emerging theory (Agar 1999).

Feedback from others

With reference to the development of self-esteem, Wells (2001) describes 'first, and most basic, is the idea of reflected appraisals, in which people learn who they are and how well they are doing through the social responses of others to them'. A basic summary suggests that receiving positive appraisals bolsters self-esteem and receiving negative appraisals reduces self-esteem (Owens *et al.* 2001). The receipt of positive and negative appraisals is also supported in the data; however, the women's receipt of negative appraisals was far more common than the receipt of positive appraisals. Some of the appraisals low-income women received during their day-to-day activities included the following:

> I did a course about five years, six years ago and I was best in the class. I did so well. Confidence went over the top. Until this guy, their father, he put me down, put me down and now, if I want to do something, I'm not confident enough. I lost that. I went down to the bottom. And [my confidence] suffered a lot.
>
> (Eva)

> I hate being on the [welfare] system. I want to get off it. I want to get out of it. And I think I have for a long, long time but I've never had the encouragement to I suppose. It's a rut. And the longer you're in the rut the longer it is to get out of it.
>
> (Lisa)

> I notice that the area where [my son] goes to school it's a fairly expensive area and the mums roll up in their big cars and their tennis skirts and they all, they're all really cliquey and a lot of them won't talk to me because I'm a single mum.
>
> (Beth)

As Poole (2000: 141) notes 'our self-concept develops through our interactions with others. If we are defined as "ugly" or "fat" or "stupid" then we may begin to see ourselves as such and behave accordingly'. Both positive and negative examples of such appraisals were evident in the data, which reinforced the women's marginalised position and contributed to their social exclusion. For example:

> Because he would put me down. 'You don't know nothing. You are dumb.'
>
> (Eva)

> And anyway we ended up, one night we had a few fights and I, I got hurt because he, because I wasn't eating properly. He was telling me that I was too fat. I was actually really underweight, but I didn't see it.
>
> (Beth)

> My mother she said 'Oh it's no good if you have children and different fathers'. And I worked very hard to keep my marriage, but he wouldn't understand it ... A couple of years ago I wanted to do the computer

course and my husband said 'Oh you're no good for that', you know. 'No good for that.' So, 'who's going to look after the kids?'

(Fiona)

These are but a few of the many ways in which women were told, and interpreted, that they were not meeting social expectations. Being told they weren't good enough represents a direct evaluation of a negative appraisal. For example, Eva was told she was dumb, Beth was told she was fat, and Fiona was told she was wrong for being a single mother, and that she was not good enough to do a computer course.

In the above instances, the women experienced stigma, which 'is associated with those inferior attributes which are commonly regarded as major norm infractions' (Page 1984: 4). In his classic work, Goffman (1963) identified three 'types' of stigma, or facets by which a person can be stigmatised. These include physical deformities, deficits in character and lineal inadequacies, which are all based upon socially accepted norms. Failure to adhere to such norms can result in stigma. The above examples, of being dumb, fat, or a single mother, all fit into the 'deficits of character' type. Unsurprisingly, stigma was also experienced by the women interviewed. As Lisa attests:

You feel trapped. And you feel a little bit isolated sometimes and you feel like you've got this stigma over you. 'Oh, single mother. Sole parent.'

Appraisals regarding these stigmatising attributes contributed to the feelings of marginalisation experienced by the women. As Cook and McCormick (2006) note, the mechanics through which people are marginalised and excluded include both the stigma associated with breaking social norms, and 'differentiation', which is the creation and maintenance of boundaries through divergent identities (Hall *et al.* 1994). While these examples demonstrate interpreting feedback as a negative indictment on character, not receiving appraisals also negatively contributed to the women's self-esteem and social exclusion.

Lack of feedback from others

Returning to one of the original two statements, for Irene, a disabled woman who lived alone, not receiving negative appraisals has made her feel 'more confident' as 'no one's judging' her. Vicky also described how her confidence improved as she moved from a wealthy suburb, where she didn't 'fit in' and was excluded, to a low-income suburb where she felt 'normal':

[Low-income Suburb]'s quite a good area to be poor in! Although there is sort of some money around, but generally people aren't as superficial. Yeah, or aren't as judgemental about that sort of thing as they are in other places. A lot of people here are the working class kind, in the suburbs.

So I don't feel, you know, that disadvantaged. Although when I lived in [High-income Suburb] before I moved over to this side of town, I did feel it a *lot* more there

(Vicky)

Irene's and Vicky's experiences are challenges to the original proposition, as no direct appraisals are being made. These examples, however, rather than dismissing the emerging theory, provide refinement on two issues: first, there is evidence of the common-sense strategy of avoiding negative appraisals (Rosenberg 1979); and second, there is evidence of generalised appraisals being perceived from others. Avoiding negative appraisals would account for Christine and Irene's withdrawal from society as they preferred to be at home, and Vicky's move to a suburb where people weren't as 'judgmental'. Generalised appraisals refer to the women feeling that they were being judged, even when no direct verbal communication was being made to them. The nature of these generalised appraisals is outlined below.

Generalised feedback from others

Analysis of the data revealed that the perception of generalised feedback from others was a common experience. Tying this to theories on self-esteem, the women's experiences reflect the concept of 'social comparison', first put forward by Festinger (1954). Here,

> 'other people provide important reference sources for calibrating social reality and anchoring self-appraisals. Social skills, attributes, and identities lack absolute value and a clear evaluative metric. Thus, other people serve as essential reference points for deciding what is normal and what is good, providing external standards by which persons can comparatively assess their own merit or value'
>
> (Wells 2001: 305–6)

Again, as with the interpretation of direct appraisals, negative generalised appraisals far outweighed positive generalised appraisals, which were effectively non-existent. The following excerpts illustrate the women's experience:

> I mean, you know, they can point their finger at me, and say I'm a sole parent and an ex-commission woman.
>
> (Prue)

> And that makes me sad to some extent, where I feel as though I always have to defend myself to someone. I mean, even though they're not asking, I see their eyes. I know what they're thinking even before they open their mouth.
>
> (Glenda)

Well, they do look down on people who get the pension ... And people do look at you, you know, like, 'Well, she thinks she's so important. We're not paying out tax to support her!'

(Carley)

In the above excerpts, demonstrating how negative appraisals were received despite no direct communication with others, the women felt they were being judged, and judged negatively. This adds weight to the presupposition that welfare stigma contributed to social exclusion, as low-income women withdrew from society to avoid the negative direct and generalised appraisals they constantly perceived.

The emerging theory, however, does not end with what women felt other people thought of them, as their withdrawal from public life was also impacted upon by what the women thought of themselves. When direct or generalised appraisals were not made by or in reference to others, the women made self-appraisals. Some examples include:

Its like I'm a lower member of society because I had a child when I was younger and we split up.

(Beth)

I mean, where do I fit in society? Just one of the many cretins just lurking about, trying to exist, I think. That's about all I can say. You don't feel very important. Just a cretin.

(Olivia)

Well, [my daughter] doesn't get to go on all the [school] excursions. And I speak to the principal and I have no pride. I am not allowed to have pride. And my husband's not allowed pride.

(Nora)

Probably the biggest deal was having to go on a single mother's pension and going and having to apply for that was sort of a big deal. I found it really embarrassing.

(Vicky)

The above quotes are examples of negatively self-perceived behaviours and attributes; such as having a child when you were young, having to apply for the pension, not being able to afford school excursions, or being a cretin. Again, these self-appraisals overlap feelings of stigma, as the negatively perceived attributes and behaviours contravene major social norms, such as having children in stable relationship at an appropriate age, being financially secure, and being a respectable person. Additionally, these self-appraisals share the assumptions of Cooley's (1902) classic conception of the 'looking glass self' where individuals imagine their appearance and the reaction of others.

In addition to the self-evaluation of attributes, behaviour and activities, the women also reflected on their social position by evaluating social symbols.

Again, sociological theories on self-esteem support this conceptualisation. Such evaluations are known as 'identification' (Wells 2001), where individuals include their association with highly regarded others or objects in their own self-concept. It has been asserted that this is especially pertinent for women, who emphasise their connectedness to others, such as being in desirable social relationships or belonging to favourable groups, as important to their own self-regard (Josephs *et al.* 1992). Such evaluations have a dynamic and recursive connection to social exclusion. Women who are marginalised, isolated or excluded may have poor self-esteem, as Eva exemplifies:

> Because you're just at home and nothing to do. You get lonely. Because I have no friends, I just go to the shop. Look after them two [children] and you know, you get lonely in a way.
>
> (Eva)

Additionally, women with poor self-esteem may not wish to socialise or connect with others, explaining Christine's depletion of self-esteem to 'the stage where I don't want to leave the house anymore' (Christine).

Below are some illustrations of identification with particular social or cultural groups and the women's self-evaluations. As can be seen, women who identified with socially valued, and hence socially included, groups or relationships, such as workers, good mothers, and those who contribute to society had more positive self-evaluations, whereas women who identified with self-perceived undesirable groups and relationships, and were thus socially excluded, such as single mothers, welfare recipients, or the disabled had more negative self-evaluations.

One explanation for such conceptions is that identifying with socially valued groups and relationships conforms to major social norms, whereas identifying with undesirable social groups and relationships contravenes major social norms, and therefore is both marginalising and attracts stigma. The following excerpts reflect this assertion, beginning with socially valued groups and relationships identified in the data, such as workers, good housekeepers, contributors to society, and good mothers:

> I think it's very good for your soul and your health and your mental health and your ability to mix with people. It's interesting and sometimes it's fun. I like working and I think it's very good to be busy. So, I think it's a good thing. It gets you up out of bed, everyday, going off. So, you feel it's very good for self-esteem and importance.
>
> (Olivia)

> I am a very good financial controller. I manage the house, bills, me, [Partner] and two kids. And the house is $200 rental a week, but still I do OK because I know how to manage my money.
>
> (Tania)

Oh, look, I mean once upon a time, it would have been, 'Oh, society's providing for me'. Whereas I feel that society should be extremely happy with me because I'm providing a great environment for my kids so they won't be social misfits. Because they've had the care and, you know, a pretty stable environment.

(Prue)

The flip-side of the above, socially valued roles, is the experience of not measuring up, of being part of a cultural group that is socially undesirable. These include the experiences of welfare recipients, single and young mothers, and the disabled, and once again, the negative experiences far outweighed the positive experiences: 'When I'm on the pension I feel like I'm no-one' (Fiona); 'I'm fed up. And I'm fed up with feeling like not being in, not contributing the way I should be. And society basically saying so' (Lisa).

I've thought about this for about two years now, three years now. If I go bankrupt then, because I'm a nothing in society pretty much, I'm a student, I'm on security, you know. I'm not managing my own business or you know, or I'm not planning to move overseas and start my whole new, you know, corporation, then I'm pretty much a no-one in society.

(Jacky)

As such, one of the most pervasive attitudes of the women interviewed was that they were 'nobodies' in society, that they didn't amount to anything, and that they were different from others in a negative way. As such, these women felt socially excluded from the mainstream that did not value them and to which they did not contribute. While some women articulated that they weren't contributing (and that such contribution amounted almost exclusively to economic or professional contribution rather than motherhood), most women talked about their life not amounting to much, or not being of much value. As such, these sentiments tie together notions of self-esteem with broader social issues that contextualise what it is to contribute, and to be of value. Additionally, this contribution is what low-income women perceived as participating in society in a socially valued way, and as such, by not participating they were socially excluded and lacking in social citizenship status. The following excerpts illustrate this point, beginning with the more obvious examples containing explicit references to contribution, and then moving on to more abstract or obscure references where women imply their experiences are of no value to themselves or society. The first excerpt, provided by Lisa, indicates that motherhood alone is an insufficient contribution. Her excerpt clearly outlines that contribution equates to financial contribution towards her son's future.

I would hope to get to that stage where I'm off [welfare]. I don't want it. I don't want to have a fifteen year old saying, 'Mum. You sat on your bum and', you know. And I want to be able to turn around and provide for my son. Say, 'Here's a nest-egg son'. Or provide for the, just be able to contribute. Just be able to contribute to the future.

(Lisa)

Similarly, Irene, a disabled woman without children, and Yvonne, a married childless woman, make appeals to the worker role as the only legitimate contribution to society:

I thought, 'yeah if I can get to two years full time [work] then I'm a real member of society ... I want to achieve something. Be regarded as legitimate by society.'

(Irene)

I still wanna keep trying and I really hope that this [plan for employment] works out, 'cause I've got no other thoughts after that. Yeah, it's just depressing for me that I've done different things and they haven't amounted to anything in this world.

(Yvonne)

Below is one woman's experience which provides a potential challenge to the emerging theory. Here, Prue's sentiments were originally similar to typical constructions of the worker role as primary. However, her attitude changes after watching news reports about the negative effects of childcare on young children. In this instance she goes against even her own assumptions regarding economic acquisition as a contribution to society and instead promotes the role of mother to be of prime importance.

But I couldn't give up the job. Then [I was injured at work] and I had the six months off work. When I went back, the news every night while I was at work was how parents with a child under six-months were returning to work which affects them for life. And I ended up doing it [returning to work] while the height of all this was on the TV. I walked into the payroll office and gave two weeks' notice. And it was such a relief when I did it. I mean this job was gunna be my, 'Oh, I'm gunna get a home out of this for my kids'. When really, you know, if I had to work those awful hours and then, I don't know, I never saw my kids ... So, isn't it better for society to help a little bit in one way, rather than to, you know?

(Prue)

Prue's example contradicts the contention that financial contribution is primary. However, the key aspect of her statement that differentiates it from Lisa's and from other women's experiences is her identification with socially accepted claims, presented through news stories on the benefits provided by stay-at-home parents. At the time of her decision to leave work, these stories legitimated motherhood as a contribution to society. Rather than dismissing my contention that what it is to contribute is socially circulated, Prue's example strengthens this argument. If social trends change to favour the primacy of parenthood over financial independence, then the stigma associated with welfare mothers would diminish. However, at present in Australian society we see a reduction in the promotion of the mother role for low-income women and a focus upon economic contribution (Cook and Marjoribanks 2005). This position is now enshrined in policy, such as the *Employment and workplace relations legislation amendment (Welfare to work and other measures) Act 2005 (No. 154)* where all single parents whose youngest child is over the age of 6 must return to work. Welfare policies, in both Australia and the United Kingdom (Cook and Marjoribanks 2005; Levitas 1998), have promoted work as a route out of social exclusion. However, in Levitas's (1998: 23) study of New Labour, the terms social exclusion and exclusion from paid work were used virtually interchangeably, 'while a similar elision occurs between "people" and "workers"'. This is, however, problematic for low-income single parents as the types of jobs low-income women are being encouraged to take up in order to improve their connection to the community typically attract low wages and lack advancement opportunities (Litt *et al.* 2000). Such marginal and problematic employment can serve to further exclude low income women as they struggle to meet the demands of both their mother and worker roles (Smith *et al.* 2000).

Conclusion

In the above analysis, two points were identified that are paramount to understanding low-income women's experience of marginalisation and social citizenship. First, self-esteem mediated the extent to which low-income women felt they wanted to venture outside their homes, and participate in society. Second, how low-income women viewed themselves depended on reflected appraisals which hinged on whether they perceived they were regarded as fulfilling a socially valued role or not. Performing a socially valued role legitimated low-income women receiving welfare benefits, as they thought of themselves as contributing to society. Not fulfilling a socially valued role stigmatised women, as they regarded themselves as not contributing. It was interesting to note that mothering was rarely regarded as a socially valued role. Instead, socially valued roles focused on work and financial contribution. The lack of respect accorded to low-income women welfare recipients de-legitimates their identities as mothers, carers, domestic workers, feminised workers and citizens. There is a need for low-income women to reclaim these identities, as is proposed by feminist scholars (see for example Lister 1997). However, as Link and Phelan (2001a) note, felt stigma typically results in strained and uncomfortable social situations with potential stigmatisers, more constricted social networks, low self-esteem, depressive symptoms and unemployment and loss of income. These challenges may make women's transition from welfare to work even more difficult.

As Calhoun (1994: 15) suggests, there needs to be a new focus on 'claiming, legitimating and valuing identities commonly suppressed or devalued by mainstream cultures'. As long as this process fails to occur, a culturally imperial situation is created, mirroring Young's (1990) fifth form of oppression. As she states, 'to experience cultural imperialism means to experience how the dominant meanings of a society render the particular perspectives of one's own group invisible at the same time as they stereotype one's group and mark it out as the Other' (Young 1990: 58–59). This experience was evidenced in the low-income women's experiences when they spoke about not feeling normal and being judged by others. While meagre welfare benefits subject low-income women to impoverished lives, failing to make ends meet and failing to provide adequately for their families reinforced stigma and shame. As such, welfare benefits, instead of providing social citizenship as is commonly understood, can be seen to perpetuate low-income women's depleted social citizenship and social exclusion. Providing low-income women with inadequate financial assistance with normative strings attached can be seen to reduce low-income women's self-esteem, echoing de Tocqueville's ([1835] 1997) claim 'the right of the poor to obtain society's help is unique in that instead of elevating the heart of the man who exercises it, it lowers him' (Goldberg 2001: 299).

What is required is a shift in attitudes towards low-income women receiving welfare benefits, to dispel pejorative conceptions of them as 'welfare cheats' and 'dole bludgers'. Additionally, increases in benefit levels, and meaningful programs and services to connect low-income women to the community with opportunities for skill development, self-esteem enhancement and self-improvement will assist women to become socially involved and better integrated into communities, enabling them to participate in the social practices other citizens take for granted.

Note

1 All names in parentheses are pseudonyms to protect the participant's identity.

2.4 Inner city high-rise living: a catalyst for social exclusion and social connectedness?

Claire Henderson-Wilson

This chapter is based on a conference paper that is to be published in the proceedings of the Australasian Housing Researchers' Conference 2008: Henderson-Wilson, C. (2009) 'Inner city high-rise living: a catalyst for social exclusion and social connectedness?', in *Refereed papers from the Australasian Housing Researchers' Conference 2008 (AHRC08)*, RMIT University Melbourne, forthcoming 2009. Permission has been granted by the publishers, RMIT, for the use of this material.

Introduction

This chapter discusses the concepts 'social exclusion' and 'social connectedness' which may result from living in inner city high-rise housing. Using data from the 'Living High But Healthy' study completed in 2006, the health and wellbeing impacts of high-rise living are explored. The chapter begins with a review of literature on high-rise living, social exclusion and social connectedness. This is followed by discussion of the 'Living High But Healthy' study findings in relation to social exclusion and social connectedness and lastly, the notion that inner city high-rise living may be a catalyst for these concepts is explored.

Inner city high-rise living in Australia

Traditionally, Australians have lived in low density, detached houses with modest sized backyards. However, since 1996 the growth of apartment living in Australia has accelerated, particularly in the major cities of Melbourne and Sydney (Australian Bureau of Statistics 2004). The trend towards high density living is common in countries such as Hong Kong and Singapore and is gaining prominence in Australia. At the beginning of the 1990s there were approximately one dozen privately owned or rented high-rise apartment buildings in the Central Business District of Melbourne and by 2003 there were over 100 (Crabb 2003). The City of Melbourne (2000) estimated that between 1996 and 2000, the number of inner city apartment dwellers in Melbourne increased almost three-fold. Similarly, Census statistics reveal that there was an increase in the proportion of multi-unit dwellings (including high-rise apartment buildings) constructed in the inner ring of the City of Sydney during the period 1995–7 (Bounds 2001). In addition to residents who privately rent or own an inner city high-rise apartment, there are some residents who live in public high-rise housing via government housing allocation, and with somewhat limited choice. Public high-rise housing traditionally resulted from the need to accommodate people living in the slums of inner city Melbourne and Sydney in the 1960s (Costello 2005). Currently, it accommodates people on limited incomes, with complex physical and psychological needs (Bartolomei *et al.* 2003; Judd *et al.* 2002; McNelis and Reynolds 2001). Public high-rise housing is often associated with social disadvantage and disorder, but recently developed privately owned and rented apartments located within the Central Business District of Melbourne and Sydney are viewed as luxurious places for the privileged (Costello 2005). The trend towards inner city apartment living has seen it promoted as a symbol of affluent living and vital for ensuring cities are economically, socially and environmentally sustainable (Costello 2005; Burton 2000).

Health implications of housing tenure

An interrogation of relevant literature suggests that housing tenure (whether or not the household owns or rents the property, and whether the property is rented in the public or private sectors) directly impacts the quality of life of residents and is associated with differing levels of mortality and morbidity. Studies reveal that mortality rates among owner-occupiers are 20–25 per cent lower than among public renters, and similar differences have been observed for morbidity rates (Filakti and Fox 1995; Gould and Jones 1996; Easterlow *et al.* 2000; Smith *et al.* 2003). Smith *et al.* (2003) suggested that there are three explanations to account for the relationship between housing tenure and poorer health. First, owner-occupation may have therapeutic or even curative properties. Second, people with poor health may find it more difficult to attain and consequently sustain home ownership and thirdly, alternatives to owning a house may be disproportionately available to people with health problems.

The public rental sector of inner city high-rise housing is often dominated by residents with health complaints and lower socio-economic status (McNelis and Reynolds 2001; Bartolomei *et al.* 2003; Judd *et al.* 2002; Randolph and Judd 2000; Apparicio and Seguin 2006), thus making home ownership unrealistic in many cases. Freeman (1993) suggested that where high-rise housing is mainly occupied by lower income residents, such residents may have had a worse than average level of health (both mental and physical) before they lived in that type of accommodation, indicating a correlative rather than causative relationship. If accessing home ownership is a way of improving people's health, it is important that inner city residents find a way to secure owner-occupancy. Smith *et al.* (2003) suggested that two key factors seem to prevent this from successfully occurring: inability to pay and finding appropriate accommodation. People with ongoing health problems often have limited incomes and increased expenses, putting extra burden on their ability to pay for housing and also to compete in the marketplace. Smith *et al.* (2003) argued that this resulting financial insecurity deters some residents from home ownership, and may compound the ill health of such people. Finding appropriate accommodation is another concern for people with poor health. The process of finding a suitable home can be rather stressful and lengthy though generally and even more so if one has a health complaint. Furthermore, tenure has been shown to influence residents' housing choice and control. Home owners can be considered to feel a sense of autonomy, security and personal identity (Elsinga and Hoekstra 2005), whilst public housing tenants may feel powerless and have limited choice.

Social exclusion and inner city high-rise living

Social exclusion can be widely applied to refer to poverty, deprivation, discrimination and inequality (Milbourne 2002). According to Cappo (2002) in VicHealth (2005: 1), 'social exclusion is the process of being shut out from the social, economic, political and cultural systems which contribute to the integration of a person into the community'. It is commonly assumed that residents of Australian public housing (including high-rise housing) are at risk of being socially excluded because they are often socioeconomically disadvantaged and experiencing low incomes and high unemployment rates (Arthurson 2004; Randolph and Holloway 2004; Baum 2003). Arthurson *et al.* (2006) revealed that by the year 2000, 89 per cent of Australian public housing tenants were receiving welfare benefits compared to approximately 20 per cent in 1966. In addition, Baum (2003), who developed a typology of Australian cities that are socially disadvantaged, suggested that public housing areas are characterised by unemployment, residential turnover and disengagement from the labour force.

Randolph and Holloway (2004) completed an analysis of socially excluded areas within Melbourne and Sydney using Census data from 1996 and 2001. An aim of their research was to see if social disadvantage is predominantly associated with living in public housing. Results indicated that in 2001, areas of Sydney and Melbourne that had high proportions of public housing were severely disadvantaged. Whilst both cities were considered to have similar levels of disadvantage, as Melbourne has a higher proportion of high-rise public housing, it was suggested that this city may experience more social exclusion (Randolph and Holloway 2004). However, the results of Randolph and Holloway's (2004) study indicated that social disadvantage is not confined to public housing and that of the one million plus residents living in areas of high disadvantage in Melbourne and Sydney in 2001, only a quarter lived in areas with high numbers of public housing. Furthermore, the results indicated that the inner city areas of Melbourne and Sydney did not account for substantial areas of social disadvantage. Randolph and

Holloway (2004) suggested that gentrification had pushed urban residents who were considered poor to middle suburban areas, except for the inner city areas containing public housing. Arthurson (2004: 268) concluded from her review of debates surrounding the redevelopment of public housing estates in Sydney that:

> In Australia as elsewhere, changes to targeting of public housing, restructuring of the welfare state, economic and industry restructuring and fiscal constraints mean that public housing is the repository for the most excluded tenants, rather than the cause of problems per se.

A negative image, or stigma of a neighbourhood, can lead to socially excluded residents. Stigma is associated with shame and disgrace and can leave residents feeling uncomfortable and unacceptable (Wassenberg 2004). Stigma is commonly experienced by residents of public high-rise housing estates despite the fact that when such developments were constructed in the 1960s and 1970s, they were considered 'highlights of modern planning' (Wassenberg 2004: 224). By labelling public housing estates as socially excluded, the term is used to identify the underlying symptoms of stigma rather than as a mechanism for understanding the process of decline. This can accentuate the stigma of public housing estates and could lead to housing policies that rather than focusing on the causes of social exclusion, focus on reducing its effects (Arthurson and Jacobs 2004). Residents of public high-rise housing estates are likely to perceive different aspects of their housing and neighbourhood in different ways, dependent on their sense of belonging. Some residents may explain stigma in reference to the irresponsible behaviour of fellow residents and to the lack of positive role models for children (Hastings 2004). Others may not feel connected to their neighbourhood and may not use community facilities (Hastings 2004). Forrest and Kearns (2001: 2135) suggested that communication between residents shapes the image of their neighbourhood and stated: 'neighbourhoods seem to acquire their identity through an on-going commentary between themselves and this continuous dialogue between different groups and agencies shapes the cognitive map of the city and establishes good and bad reputations.'

One way public housing estates can overcome stigma and social exclusion is through renewal and regeneration programs. Programs such as the Neighbourhood Renewal initiative adopted in Victoria are aimed at improving public housing (including high-rise), through demolition of old estates or refurbishment, and they involve upgrading community infrastructure, including green spaces (Wassenberg 2004; Department of Human Services 2002). Having knowledge of estates may reduce the likelihood of stigma and social exclusion being associated with resident characteristics (Hastings 2004; Randolph and Judd 2000). However, as Wassenberg (2004: 229) noted, urban renewal programs are only effective if the reality changes too as in some cases: 'the old negative reputation proves to be persistent, and after some years everything looks the same as before.' In addition to renewal and regeneration programs, policies are required to deal with social exclusion. Baum (2003) suggested that initiatives are required that engage the communities experiencing social exclusion, and they need to provide flexible ways of regenerating the neighbourhoods that have regard for the multi-layered nature of disadvantage. Arthurson and Jacobs (2003, 2004) suggested that policies aimed at reducing social exclusion need to focus on all housing tenures, rather than just public housing. Furthermore, Lawrence (2005) suggested that policy decision makers, social science researchers and urban design professionals should use a range of quantitative and qualitative analysis methods in order to enhance their understanding of the social and cultural dimensions of housing developments. Judd and Randolph (2006) supported Lawrence's (2005) view and proposed that qualitative analysis methods can be applied to gain a deeper understanding of the social and behavioural dimensions associated with public housing renewal.

Social connectedness and inner city high-rise living

A sense of social connectedness can be achieved through effective social capital and social cohesion. 'Social capital' has a range of different definitions and interpretations, but is commonly defined as 'networks between people that lead to cooperation and beneficial outcomes. Trust is also seen as central to the successful operation of these networks' (Baum and Palmer 2002: 352). Social capital forms a subset of 'social cohesion' as it refers to the social structures that facilitate the actions of members within a community (Kawachi and Berkman 2000). 'Social cohesion' therefore refers to two intertwined features of communities, these are: i) the absence of latent social conflict (e.g. in the form of income inequality, racial tensions or social polarisation) and ii) the presence of strong social bonds (measured by levels of social capital, i.e. trust and social norms) (Kawachi and Berkman 2000). There are at least three ways in which social capital can affect the health of urban communities. First, social capital may influence the health behaviours of residents through promotion of health information and exertion of control over negative health-related behaviour (Kawachi and Berkman 2000). A second way social capital can affect the health of residents is through access to local services and amenities (Kawachi and Berkman 2000). If residents have access to public transport, community health services and recreational facilities, their health and wellbeing may be enhanced. A final way that social capital may affect residents' health is through the processes of providing psychosocial support and acting as a source of mutual respect and self-esteem (Kawachi and Berkman 2000).

How urban developments (including high-rise buildings) are designed can influence the social capital and sense of social connectedness amongst residents. For instance, Leyden (2003) completed a study on the relationship between urban design and social capital and found that residents who lived in mixed-use developments with opportunities for walking rather than driving as a mode of transport (i.e. sustainable developments), had a higher level of social capital and social cohesion than those who lived in developments lacking these features. Conversely, high density high-rise developments can reduce social connectedness amongst residents as there are limited opportunities for them to participate in spontaneous and short-term activities (i.e. eating outside private apartments and playing sport or games) and the large volume of people may result in some residents withdrawing and refusing to participate in community activities (Williams 2005; Adams 1992). However, the social connectedness of urban high-rise developments may influence residential satisfaction. Halpern (1995) suggested that if people are in frequent contact with their neighbours, then the objective quality of their house makes little difference to their level of residential satisfaction. On the other hand, Halpern (1995) asserted that if people are not in frequent contact with their neighbours then consequently, the objective quality of their house has a large impact on their satisfaction. In other words, 'residents who are involved in their local community tend to be happy with where they live regardless of the physical quality of their homes' (Halpern 1995: 113).

Baum and Palmer (2002) found, from their study of residents' perceptions of the influence of place on levels of social capital, that there exists a direct link between urban infrastructure and social capital. These authors concluded that higher levels of social capital are likely to occur in neighbourhoods where residents have a positive image of their environment and where their environments are green with open spaces. This finding was supported by Kweon *et al.* (1998) who found that elderly public high-rise housing residents' sense of community was stronger when they spent time in outdoor green common spaces (areas with trees and grass). Additionally, natural features and open spaces were found to facilitate a sense of community in new urbanist communities (Kim and Kaplan 2004) and amongst residents living in socio-economically disadvantaged areas of California (Altschuler *et al.* 2004). As well as green spaces contributing to urban neighbourhoods' social connectedness, pets have been found to facilitate social capital too. A study completed by Wood *et al.* (2005) investigated the role that pets can play in promoting social capital, by surveying a random sample of 339 Australian residents. These authors found that pets promote opportunities for their owners to have social contact with other pet owners, neighbours and members of their community. Furthermore, pets were found to motivate owners to participate in community events and to make use of community facilities (Wood *et al.* 2005).

In summary, a review of relevant literature indicates that inner city high-rise living may be a catalyst for social exclusion and social connectedness as a result of housing tenure, resident characteristics, design features and access to nature. The next section of this chapter will discuss the 'Living High But Healthy' study.

Living High But Healthy study

The 'Living High But Healthy' (LHBH) exploratory study was conducted to research the impacts of inner city high-rise living on residents' health and wellbeing. The study's data collection was conducted in 2004–5 using a mixed methods research design comprised of two phases. Phase 1 (survey phase) involved surveying 221 high-rise residents to discover the impacts of high-rise living on quality of life. In Phase 2 of the study (interview phase), semi-structured face-to-face interviews were conducted with 30 of the surveyed participants to explore the relationships between variables identified in Phase 1 of the study more deeply. The participants of the study varied in gender, age, socio-economic status, tenure (owner occupiers, private tenants or public housing tenants), geographic location (inner city Melbourne or Sydney) and proximity to natural environments (categorised as having either 'good' or 'poor' access to nature). The findings from Phase 1 of the study were statistically analysed to determine relationships between variables. The findings from Phase 2 of the study were thematically analysed to develop key themes. A final process of data analysis involved integrating the findings from both phases of the study in order to develop a synthesised set of key themes.

The next section of this chapter discusses some of the key findings of the LHBH study in relation to social exclusion and social connectedness.

Findings related to social exclusion

Phase 1 (survey phase) of the LHBH study did not collect data on the impacts of social exclusion on participants' quality of life. Therefore, the findings from Phase 2 (interview phase) added richness to the data and indicated that regardless of housing tenure, participants living in high-rise housing are subject to stigma and stereotyping which may be components of social exclusion, but do not define it per se. For example, many participants had been subjected to derogatory comments relating to living in high-rise housing, including both those who owned or privately rented their apartment and those who lived in public housing. Many of the residents, particularly public housing tenants, shared concerns about living in a socially exclusive neighbourhood and desired a more harmonious and inclusive environment. For instance, one participant who lived in public housing commented: 'I don't know if it's that we're treated like second class citizens because we're in public housing, or the people in public housing are truly second class. Like I don't see myself as being less than or more than anybody else you know?' Stigma associated with living in high-rise housing was also expressed by a number of the residents (from all tenures). For example, a participant who owned her high-rise apartment mentioned: 'because sometimes I get that sense of, you know people say "well I live in a unit" in a kind of derogative way, like it's second to a house or whatever, but I guess it depends on your family situation too whether you've got a partner or whether you've got kids but as a single person I really wouldn't want to live anywhere else … '

Social exclusion is commonly experienced by residents of public housing who often live in socially disadvantaged areas (Arthurson 2004; Randolph and Holloway 2004; Baum 2003). However, the findings of this project indicate that elements of social exclusion such as stigma and stereotyping, are not just affecting public housing tenants; residents who own and privately rent their apartment also feel stigmatised and stereotyped by their community. The findings imply that although residents who own or privately rent their inner city apartments may have better living conditions than their public housing counterparts, they too are subject to stigma and stereotyped images of apartment dwellers. The findings reinforce the view of Forrest and Kearns (2001) who suggested that dialogue between different groups and agencies shapes the image of the city (and high-rise living) and establishes good and bad reputations. Tenure is synonymous with stigma and stereotyping which may be components of social exclusion, but do not define it per se and contribute to residents' quality of life. Tenure differences accounted for residents' satisfaction with their design and development, sense of social connectedness and choice and control. Significantly, and perhaps not surprisingly, residents who own and privately rent their apartment were found to have higher levels of wellbeing than residents who publicly rent their apartment. This finding concurs with previous research and indicates that there appears to be a direct relationship between wellbeing and tenure (Hiscock *et al.* 2003; Macintyre *et al.* 2003; Smith *et al.* 2003; Sooman and Macintyre 1995). Furthermore, owning or privately renting a home may increase health promoting characteristics such as self-esteem and independence (Waters 2001).

Findings related to social connectedness

The findings from Phase 1 (survey phase) of the LHBH study indicated that the participants' satisfaction with their sense of social connectedness varied according to their tenure. The findings from Phase 2 (interview phase) supported the findings from Phase 1 and indicated that participants' sense of social connectedness varied from non-existent to strong depending on their tenure. For example, participants who owned their apartment typically felt their development had a strong sense of community, as represented by this participant's quote: 'we try and create consciously on our part, we particularly with people we know, have this kind of open house gathering on a Sunday night.' Residents' social connectedness was influenced by their tenure, access to natural environments and the design of their development. Where developments were appropriately designed to accommodate resident gatherings and opportunities for residents to entertain, social connectedness was fostered. Functioning social networks and a strong sense of social capital were found to be important predictors of residents' enhanced wellbeing. Many residents felt their development lacked a strong sense of social connectedness being due to the short-term rental market and the fact that they were not able to access outdoor areas to entertain. The inclusion of useable open spaces (preferably with barbecue facilities) was found to create a stronger sense of community within high-rise developments. For example, one participant mentioned: 'generally I would say that it would be lovely to have a useable outdoor space with a barbeque you could invite friends over and socialise in the outdoor space that would be lovely ... ' This reinforces the assertion of Baum and Palmer (2002) and indicates that social capital is likely to occur where residents have opportunities to access green open spaces. However, for many residents with poor access to nature, such opportunities were not available, or were not safely accessible.

On the other hand, a number of residents felt that their development had a strong sense of social connectedness due to proactive residents who had introduced formal gatherings, support networks and community newsletters. Thus, the findings concur with Halpern (1995) and indicate that residents who are involved in their local community are happy with where they live regardless of the design of their homes. As there were few pet owners studied, the findings are limited as to the role pets can play in promoting social capital (Wood *et al.* 2005). The findings do suggest that if more residents had pets, there could be more opportunities for a stronger sense of social connectedness to be created within developments. However, this means that high-rise developments need to be appropriately designed to cater for pets and housing management bodies need to allow residents to own pets.

Inner city high-rise living: a catalyst for social exclusion and social connectedness?

The LHBH study findings suggest that inner city high-rise living may indeed be a catalyst for social exclusion and social connectedness. On the one hand, high-rise living may leave some residents (particularly public housing residents) feeling socially excluded as a result of their housing form and tenure. On the other hand, high-rise living provides many residents with opportunities for social connectedness. To create more socially inclusive public high-rise housing estates, various initiatives can be implemented. For instance, the 'Redfern/ Waterloo Partnerships Program' (NSW Government 2004) is an urban renewal initiative that involves a whole-of-government approach between the New South Wales Department of Housing, the Attorney General's Department, NSW Health, Department of Corrective Services, Department of Education and Training, Department of Aboriginal Affairs, Department of Community Services, NSW Police, Department of Infrastructure, Planning and Natural Resources, the Roads Traffic Authority and the Department of Ageing, Disability and Home Care. The strategy aims to redevelop the existing high-rise housing in Redfern and Waterloo, to ensure more appropriate and safe housing is available to residents, to foster an inclusive and cohesive community, to minimise drug and alcohol abuse and to provide residents with education and employment opportunities.

Social connectedness can be strengthened in inner city high-rise developments through community development initiatives such as community and
rooftop gardens, cultural events, special interest groups and informal restaurant
gatherings. For example, the Atherton Gardens public high-rise housing estate
in Fitzroy, Melbourne, introduced a community choir to strengthen community ties amongst its ethnically diverse group of residents (Whinnett 2005).
Additionally, community gardens provide residents with an opportunity to
interact with a range of people. Such initiatives could be introduced in all
inner city high-rise housing developments to develop a strong sense of social
connectedness and to create a more socially inclusive urban environment.

2.5 The influence of 'access' on social exclusion and social connectedness for people with disabilities

Janet Owens

Social exclusion of people with disabilities has been a focus of governments, communities, service providers and by people with disabilities themselves over the last few decades. While marginalisation of this group is well recognised it has been difficult to clarify the relationship between the intertwined material, political and social elements that create a social divide (Bowe 1978). Addressing these elements is critical in order for people with disabilities to participate equally in society. Millar (2007) has suggested that participation is synonymous with social inclusion and connectedness but achieving participation has been problematic for many people with disabilities. Access is a concept that is increasingly used as a bridge between structural and social variables and participation outcomes and this is evidenced in human rights instruments, legislation and policies. Regardless of this, access barriers persist. A better understanding of the mechanics and influences on access, and of how access as a phenomenon is achieved or denied, could contribute to solutions and social inclusion. In this chapter, an understanding of access for people with disabilities is sought through a qualitative analysis of the literature.

Disability and social exclusion

Disability is a multi-dimensional concept. Historically, the term 'disability' has been applied to people in society who have impairments or bodily differences (Williams 2001; Barnes and Mercer 2006) and as a personal tragedy for the person with impairment (Oliver 1996). This view is evident in the medical model of disability, where disability is conceptualised as biomedical difference (Williams 2001).

In contrast, the social model of disability asserts that social, cultural, political and economic factors oppress and exclude (Oliver 1996), regardless of a person's impairment. The dynamic relationship between structural factors which affect participation, the person and their personal characteristics, and limitations they have in performing activities are now widely considered to contribute to the experience of disability (World Health Organisation 2002).

In an early discussion on access, Bowe (1978) determined that people with disabilities were handicapped by social, environmental, architectural and transportation barriers and by the social divides that these barriers create. More recently, the relationship of these dimensions were recognised by Scheer *et al.* (2003: 228) as 'a web of barriers' that compromise access and social inclusion. Toward addressing these barriers, Finkelstein (1993) inferred that access was the missing ingredient for living from day to day in the physical world. He suggested that 'enabling justice' was required for people with disabilities, achievable through meeting material needs, having cultural respect and political participation, and enjoying socio-spatial inclusion. A similar cumulation of access was recommended by Galvin (2004: 347) as physical access to public spaces and 'contestation of attitudes and cultural imagery which devalue disabled people so they can access more positive identities'.

Access

Access is an important concept in discussions of independence, participation and social inclusion for people with disabilities (Galvin 2004; Frantz *et al.* 2006). The dimensions of access for people with disabilities have been considered in reference to specific contexts e.g. access to health care (Aday and Anderson 1981); access to rehabilitation (Heinemann 2007) and access to information technology (McKenzie 2007).

In an early investigation of access to health care, Aday and Anderson (1981) introduced the concepts of potential and realised access. Potential access focused on person and service characteristics related to structures and processes. Realised access comprised measurable indicators such as time and type of service, and subjective indicators related to consumer satisfaction. Further investigation of these aspects and applicability of the terminology could enrich our understanding of access and its role in social inclusion.

Method

A database search on EbscoHost, Academic Search Premier, CINAHL and PsychInfo resulted in a rich source of articles for analysis. Search terms included variations of: access, disability, health, rehabilitation, transportation, mobility, environment, space, geography, architecture, employment, recreation, communication, telecommunications, education, computer, Internet, assistive technology (AT), policy, legislation, sexuality, social, ageing, children, adolescent and adult.

Inclusion criteria requirements included peer reviewed full papers dated between 2001 and 2007 that reported empirical research or included social or political commentary. There were no restrictions on geographic or cultural contexts. Articles that did not focus on disability and access, had no author information or were editorials, news articles, brief commentaries or of excessive length were excluded. A total of 195 articles were identified in the database search with 159 of them meeting inclusion criteria. A selection of these articles has been used in this literature analysis.

Articles were reviewed sentence by sentence. Text that represented any latent meaning related to *access* (e.g. definition, barriers, rights to, factors contributing to) was extracted for coding. Various qualitative strategies such as category construction and mapping were used to explore the dimensions, conditions, interactions, and the evolvement of these in the data (Strauss and Corbin 1998). To establish reliability in coding, text from 10 per cent of articles was analysed by two coders who achieved 90 per cent agreement after earlier coding results were discussed and differences resolved (Miles and Huberman 1994). Validity was established through analytic induction and use of the constant comparative method for exploration of similarities, differences and emerging patterns and themes (Silverman 2001).

Results

This literature analysis has revealed a growing awareness of the facilitators of access and societal responsibilities associated with these. However, considerable access issues prevail for people with disabilities. Access is influenced by the processes through which participation is achieved and by the numerous social and structural barriers that compromise participation.

Benefits are positive outcomes of access. Benefits are demonstrated through social, educational, vocational and community participation and through the availability and ease of use of technology and infrastructure. Examples of benefits include: increased social esteem by involvement with others who display positive attitudes (McDougall *et al.* 2004; Wilson 2004); use of inclusive transport systems designed to be accessible to everyone (Barrett *et al.* 2003) and increased community participation through inclusion at school and in community gathering places (Russell 2003; Villa *et al.* 2003).

Barriers are obstacles to achievement of one's goals. Social barriers are significant in that they affect an individual's social-emotional state and sense of exclusion or inclusion (Lee and Mittelstaedt 2004). These barriers may be produced subtly and are most evident by the way people feel or behave. Structural barriers are identified through analysis of the effects of the environment, infrastructure, equipment and service provision, economics, and legislation and policy, and the relationships between these, as they impact on access for people with disabilities.

The themes that have evolved through analysis of the literature have been identified as dimensions of access. The themes are: intent; practice; context and accessibility; economic; and personal. These areas overlap to varying degrees. The analysis addresses the importance of these dimensions to the process of achieving access but also highlights the barriers that persist and solutions for these.

Intent

The theme of intent comprises of the attitudes and purpose(s) of others that become apparent through behaviour. Knowledge and awareness, which influence attitudes, contributes to intent. Human rights instruments, government, legislation and policy are structural foundations and drivers of intent; these are also included in this theme.

Reference to negative attitudes and behaviours toward people with disabilities in the literature is notable. Negative attitudes are felt to develop over time or to reflect naivety (Crawshaw 2002; C. Thomas 2004; Wilson 2004). Examples of these include: fear of disability (Barrett *et al.* 2003); lack of valuing people (Imrie 2003; C. Thomas 2004; Wilson 2004); prejudice and discrimination (McDougall *et al.* 2004; Wilson 2004; Brostrand 2006; Parish and Huh 2006); and limited expectations of people (Smith *et al.* 2004; C. Thomas 2004; Chouniard and Crooks 2005; Brostrand 2006). Negative attitudes manifest in negative behaviours such as ignoring, speaking to people with disabilities in demeaning ways or not repairing communication breakdown (Barrett *et al.* 2003; Smart 2004).

Knowledge and awareness of disability influence intent. Lack of awareness of people's daily experiences and accessibility requirements contribute to lack of expertise in service providers (Barrett *et al.* 2003; Wilson 2004; Brostrand 2006; Frantz *et al.* 2006; Parish and Huh 2006). Awareness can be influenced by training and lack of this contributes to unnecessary barriers, compromising service provision (C. Thomas 2004; Frantz *et al.* 2006; Palley 2006).

Human rights instruments, legislation and policy provide intent and influence attitudes and awareness. The enjoyment of human rights and social justice is recognised as a significant issue for people with disabilities. When one's rights are violated, human rights instruments and non-discrimination legislation can be invoked. However, people's awareness of their rights and information on these can be problematic (Barrett *et al.* 2003; Loughlin *et al.* 2004). Regardless of entitlements to human rights, inaccessibility continues to exclude people with disabilities (Barrett *et al.* 2003).

Intent is linked to practice. Government recognises the relationship between inclusive attitudes and non-discriminatory practices and society's responsibility to respond to legislation and human rights instruments (Butler *et al.* 2002). The importance of involving service users with disabilities in the development of inclusive policies, practices and services is also acknowledged by government (Palley 2006).

Legislation formalises government's stance on access and accommodation of people with disabilities. Informed practice and service provision can result from legislated requirements for policy development; in turn, policy and legislation can be influenced by examples of successful inclusive programs and can be evaluated for currency (Villa *et al.* 2003). Although legislation creates an awareness of accessibility, there may be variability in how legislation is enacted, resulting in differences of compliance, effectiveness and efficiency (Imrie 2003).

Policy can facilitate strategy development for participation and inclusion (Bigby and Balandin 2005). Barriers occur when policies are developed without input from people with disabilities or when they are not reviewed for compliance with legislation (Crawshaw 2002; Barrett *et al.* 2003; Smith *et al.* 2004). Lack of policies, or underdeveloped policies, can also compromise accessibility, service delivery and economic considerations for people with disabilities (Villa *et al.* 2003; Wilson 2004; Parish and Huh 2006; Heinemann 2007).

Key solutions for addressing intent-related barriers focus on creating positive attitude change through increased awareness (with strategic and systematic training, information, practice and policy) (McDougall 2004; Brostrand 2006) and increased occasions to engage with people with disabilities (Wilson 2004). Advocacy also contributes to increased awareness (Parish and Huh 2006). Policy initiatives ideally include disability impact statements (Russell 2003), requirements for empirical evidence (Parish and Huh 2006) and accessibility policies for professional practice and environments (Bigby and Balandin 2005).

Practice

This theme includes practitioner skills, service delivery practices and systemic issues that impact on participation. Provision of information is a practice that can enhance or impede access to services and is also considered in this theme.

Practice barriers are grounded in inadequacy of skills to effectively provide support and a comprehensive service to people with a disability (Chouniard and Crooks 2005; Frantz *et al.* 2006; Parish and Huh 2006). Unwillingness to provide a service to some people with disabilities demonstrates how practices can be influenced by intent (Minden *et al.* 2004).

Service providers create barriers when services are not fully accessible (Crawshaw 2002) or are unresponsive to identified accessibility issues (Anderson 2001). Problems are also caused when programs and practices lead to decreased access (Villa *et al.* 2003; Chouniard and Crooks 2005) or there is inadequate consultation with people with disabilities, particularly by managers (Barrett *et al.* 2003; Brostrand 2006).

Systemic barriers associated with service delivery are also evident. Poor awareness of accessibility issues throughout an organisation is indicative of inadequate systemic support and lack of training (Wilson 2004). Lack of coordination of services or gaps in services can lead to a poor response by service providers (Barrett *et al.* 2003; Russell 2003). Lack of enforcement of accessibility regulations by management can also compromise access (Barrett *et al.* 2003). These barriers result in insufficient opportunities for participation because of lack of attention to (in)accessibility, responsiveness and service coordination.

Creation of accessible information is a skill. Information barriers are created when there is lack of appropriate and relevant content (Barrett *et al.* 2003; Llewellyn 2007) and lack of accessible or alternative formats with information on where to locate these (Barrett *et al.* 2003; Frantz *et al.* 2006; Schaefer 2006). As a result, people with disabilities may have difficulty finding information or may find it inaccessible (McMillen and Soderberg 2002).

Practice-related solutions focus on several areas. Information needs to be relevant and provided accessibly in regard to content and location (Schaefer

2006). Facilitation of practitioner skill development, through training, should provide flexibility, inclusive practices and maximisation of opportunities for community participation (Barrett *et al.* 2003; McDougall *et al.* 2004; Smart 2004; Bigby and Balandin 2005). Consultation and collaboration with people with disabilities should underpin inclusive service provision and provide validation of practices that are user focused (Crawshaw 2002; P. Thomas 2004 Llewellyn 2007); these should be manager-driven. In addition, managers should oversee the developments of inclusive policies and initiatives to support community capacity building (Brostrand 2006; Palley 2006).

Context and accessibility

The theme of context and accessibility includes the different environments in which the processes of access occur as well as provisions for ease of use and accommodations for people. This theme comprises design, physical, spatial, temporal and technological factors, all of which are underpinned by accessibility, the extent to which products, spaces, places and services are available for use to the broadest group of people. While considerable progress has been made in achieving user-friendly environments, numerous barriers still exist.

Design practices affect use and poor design compromises access to landscaped and built environments and to contents, technology and transportation systems (Tamm and Prellwitz 2001; Barrett *et al.* 2003; Imrie 2003; P. Thomas 2004). Accessibility outcomes related to design are also affected by the minimum requirements that manufacturers and builders must meet; however, these may not provide a satisfactory degree of access for the user (Schaefer 2006). Universal design principles which have been developed to provide access for all are also not being routinely applied at the design stage (Butler *et al.* 2002).

Physical barriers pertain to built environments and modes of transportation. Some examples of these are: inaccessible buildings and contents (P. Thomas 2004); inaccessible automatic teller machines and countertops in banks (McMillen and Soderberg 2002), and unsatisfactory provision of different transport modes, such as maxi taxis for accommodating people in wheelchairs (Barrett *et al.* 2003; Smith *et al.* 2004).

Spatial barriers create inequalities in the way people move through environments and plan their activities (Chouniard and Crooks 2005). Spatial barriers include: poor organisation of parking lots and public toilets (Imrie 2003); poor conditions of streets and parks; inaccessible locations of signage and timetable information; limited space to accommodate wheelchair users (Barrett *et al.* 2003; Wilson 2004); conditions imposed by sand and snow on mobility (Tamm and Prellwitz 2001); and distance required to travel to service providers (Smith *et al.* 2004).

Time also contributes to access. Delays in providing information, implementing services, providing adequate timeframes for people with disabilities to complete activities, and delays in responding to people who are experiencing accessibility issues are temporal barriers that contribute to information, practice and service barriers (Barrett *et al.* 2003; P. Thomas 2004; Wilson 2004). Requirements for time can also result in costs; an example is costs for the additional time required to accommodate a person and wheelchair when using a taxi (Barrett *et al.* 2003).

Also related to context are technologies and resources that people may require. For many people, assistive technology (AT) is essential for maximising function and participation. The lack of availability of AT or lack of technology in particular settings can result in lack of opportunity (Russell 2003; Smith *et al.* 2004). Since appropriate selection and evaluation of AT is reliant on trained staff, lack of these human resources adversely affects use of AT (Smart 2004; Wilson 2004).

Solutions for context and accessibility should focus initially on application of universal design principles and user-centred design practices for flexible and cost-effective solutions (Anderson 2001; Schaefer 2006). In addition, in physical and spatial environments there should be full, effective and early response to accessibility requirements and standards (Barrett *et al.* 2003; P. Thomas 2004; Bigby and Balandin 2005). The time requirements of people with disabilities need to be incorporated into program development and community activities (Crawshaw 2002; Palley 2006). Use of AT is critical for participation and quality of life for many people with disabilities; these resources, as well as computer access, should be provided as required (Scheer *et al.* 2003; Bigby and Balandin 2005). In addition, there must be people who support the use and maintenance of equipment and have particular skills in these areas (Villa *et al.* 2003).

Personal

This theme includes a range of factors that relate to the person and their engagement in access. These factors include gender (being female) (C. Thomas 2004; Parish and Huh 2006); aging (Minden *et al.* 2004); and cultural diversity (Putnam *et al.* 2003). Personal factors also include activity restrictions which may be related to impairment or be socially imposed (C. Thomas 2004). Examples cited in the literature are poor comprehension of information (Wilson 2004); illiteracy (Parish and Huh 2006; McKenzie 2007); and lack of concentration or limited communication and social skills (Wilson 2004; Bigby and Balandin 2005). Addressing these aspects involves awareness and attitude change and may involve practices and resources that facilitate skill development in the person.

Economic

This theme includes monetary resources, costs to individuals, cost of services and extent of comprehensive funding. People with disabilities are one of the largest minority groups to experience poverty (Parish and Huh 2006). Therefore, additional costs or lack of funding creates additional burdens. The cost of a product or service, or additional costs for procuring disability-specific products or services, means that AT, transportation, higher education, and medical and therapeutic services may be inaccessible for many people with disabilities (Barrett *et al.* 2003; Galvin 2004; Smith *et al.* 2004; Parish and Huh 2006). Budgets and criteria for funding schemes may impact on acquisition of AT (Hammel and Finlayson 2003) or assistance with independent living (Butler *et al.* 2002; Russell 2003; P. Thomas 2004). At a service level, lack of comprehensive funding of programs and community activities, or lack of integration of funding across departments to meet accessibility standards, frequently impacts on service provision and access for the person (Butler *et al.* 2002; P. Thomas 2004).

Discussion

Access is a process as well as an outcome. The use of the terms 'potential' and 'realised' access (Aday and Anderson 1981) has been revised in light of this study's outcomes. Realised access is interpreted as the achievement of an access goal, resulting in participation. As suggested by Aday and Anderson (1981), realised access is measurable; however, the inclusion of satisfaction as a subjective indicator of access may be more indicative of the psychological response to experiences at potential access points. Potential access is interpreted as occurring at each necessary point along the journey towards realised access, during which the person has either a positive experience or encounters barriers. For example, access to computer equipment in the workplace may require a response from service providers in the selection and setup of AT, followed by technical support in the workplace. Funding for AT may need to be applied for and timeframes discussed. Social interaction would occur between individuals as these events take place. At each (potential access) point, a positive or negative experience contributes to the experience of attaining realised access.

This analysis has highlighted the relationship of social and structural factors that are within and between dimensions of access. As an example, intent, which manifests in a range of practices, can be influenced by increased awareness through training. Provision of training is impacted by provision of economic resources for this purpose and by professional practices and values. Structural influences such as legislation and policy can be driving forces in creating awareness and are an impetus for compliance from service providers. Intent is further demonstrated through design practices for an accessible world and for provision of resources for successful participation.

While the role of the personal dimension in access is recognised (C. Thomas 2004), the impact of personal factors is noted in the literature to a far lesser extent than barriers created by social and structural factors. Regardless of an increased understanding of accessibility, community inclusion and empowerment, the social and structural barriers cited by Bowe (1978) continue to challenge access and social inclusion for people with disabilities (McMillen and Soderberg 2002; Barrett *et al.* 2003; Brostrand 2006).

The impact of these barriers are those reflected in the social model of disability, where barriers oppress and disenfranchise people with disability, impact on agency and reflect inequitable power relations (Oliver 2006; McKenzie 2007).

The limitations of this analysis are that it reflects an interpretation of authors' contributions to the literature only. The literature is not necessarily representative of the views of people with disabilities, who are primary stakeholders in the discussion and debate about the processes and outcomes of access.

Conclusion

Access is necessary for achievement of social connectedness. Access opens the door to numerous life opportunities and to exercising of agency in pursuing life goals. As an inclusive concept, access is more than gaining entry, exiting or making use of and having the right to do these, which are reflective of normative, ableist views, where the enjoyment of, and responsibility for, access is primarily dependent on agency. Access involves positive engagement and response at every process point so that equality of opportunity is realised. This involves social and political responsibility for addressing barriers that continue to impede access for people with disabilities. An inclusive concept of access should include reference to terms such as 'provision for' and 'accommodation' to reflect the social and structural response that is required.

Additional research is required to understand better the influences and processes of access. Investigation of attitudes and attitude change and how these impact on, or result from, practices is indicated and would be valuable for addressing social and structural barriers. Understanding the mechanisms used for effective consumer consultation and how to implement these would also address a number of barriers. Clarification of how barriers in each dimension impact on each other, and the consequences of these for the person and their satisfaction, would serve to 'untangle the web' and create an effective platform for social, political and economic response, all of which are required for realisation of social inclusion.

2.6 The relationship between undertaking an informal caring role and social exclusion

Sally Savage and Nicole Carvill

The aim of this chapter is to demonstrate the relationship between undertaking an informal caring role and social exclusion. There is a substantial body of literature available on the impact of caring on informal caregivers; however this literature focuses largely on identifying and measuring the impact of the caring role. The negative impact of caring is clear. A recent survey of over 4,000 carers in Australia reported that they had the lowest collective wellbeing of any group surveyed (Cummins *et al.* 2007). Differences in wellbeing between carers as a group, and non-carers, were reported in the Victorian Carers Program, a population-based study (Schofield *et al.* 1998). Carers reported less life satisfaction, less positive affect, more negative affect and greater overload compared with non-carers, regardless of age or marital status. More than one-quarter of the 945 carers in the Victorian Carers Program self-rated their health as fair or poor (Schofield *et al.* 1998) in comparison with 16 per cent of 25,900 Australians in the general population who rated their health as fair or poor in a National Health Survey (Australian Institute of Health and Welfare, 2006). In this chapter we argue that the type of exclusion experienced as a result of caregiving is not a static phenomenon, and that exclusion can be primarily social, financial, or systemic.

A carer or caregiver is someone who is unpaid and provides regular and ongoing assistance and support (physical or emotional) for a person with a physical and/or intellectual disability, mental illness or is frail aged. The person for whom they care is referred to as a care recipient. The number of people in a caring role is growing in Australia due to the ageing population and to people with disabilities living longer.

The data included in this chapter comes from several studies conducted with carers in the Barwon-South West region of Victoria for various projects. In-depth interviews were conducted with: 41 parents of a child aged up to 13 years with a disability (Jones *et al.* 2003); 77 carers in the areas of aged care, disability and mental illness (Carvill 2008); 42 parents and family carers of adolescents with a disability (Fennessy *et al.* 2008); and telephone interviews conducted with 142 community-dwelling women aged 70 or over (Ulvestad 2006). The words of the carers interviewed for these projects are used to illustrate points in this chapter.

Exclusion is not static

The situation of carers illustrates that social exclusion is not static; it can occur suddenly, and to anyone. The exclusion experienced by carers is not due to stable factors such as socioeconomic status, geographic location or race, but results from a change in specific circumstances. This type of exclusion can happen to anyone, for example when a partner or parent becomes increasingly frail or develops dementia, when a child with a disability is born, or when a family member becomes disabled due to an accident.

For some people, the change experienced on becoming a carer affects all aspects of their life, as the following comments made by older carers demonstrate:

> I've given up my life, my free time, my whole way of life. I've gone from easy going and relaxed to on the go and never stopping.
>
> (Carvill 2008: 268)

> I can't visit friends. I can't go to the craft show. I can't get out of the house. I've given everything up. Your life stops and his life stops too.
>
> (Carvill 2008: 268)

Some carers comment on specific activities that they are no longer able to do, since taking on a caring role. They are no longer able to participate in a range of activities including volunteering and physical activity:

> [My] husband's health limits activity – now cannot do Meals on Wheels, [or] go out.
>
> (Ulvestad 2006: 35)

> I used to go to the gym in the morning but I've stopped because he needs help with breakfast.
>
> (Carvill 2008: 269)

Thus, many aspects of the previous life of carers may be changed as a result of taking on a caregiving role. Important social connections and health-enhancing activities may no longer be possible.

Social exclusion

An important mechanism of exclusion for carers relates to social exclusion. Some reported that their social network had reduced significantly since the care recipient's diagnosis, resulting in a sense of social isolation. Many carers described a 'loss of freedom and spontaneity' associated with the caring role which results in social and lifestyle restrictions (Carvill 2008). Such restrictions have the potential to adversely impact on other areas of a carer's life and result in stress proliferation. The term stress proliferation is used to highlight the interaction between various stressors and to illustrate how potential lifestyle restrictions associated with caring have the potential to affect other areas of a carer's life (e.g. employment opportunities, family and peer relationships). Socioemotional support appears to improve carer wellbeing. Socioemotional support is conceptualised as the strength of the connection between the carer and their social network and is measured by a carer's perception of the availability of someone who helps them to feel good and the presence of a confidant. Conversely, carer perceptions of insufficient social support has been found to be predictive of depression and higher levels of burden for carers of a person with a mental illness (Magliano *et al.* 1998; Song *et al.* 1997). The following quotes are from carers with an aged care recipient:

> The contact that we used to have socially has gone. I'm more isolated but if people came to visit I could cope [with the role].
>
> (Carvill 2008: 272)

> I don't have as much contact with my family and friends as I used to. I miss it.
>
> (Carvill 2008: 272)

Some carers commented that the social contact they do have is with a new group of people – professional carers. Thus their social contact is linked with their caring role:

> I now have social contact with nurses and respite workers.
>
> (Carvill 2008: 272).

Parents who are caring for a child with a disability have expressed similar experiences:

> I haven't got my own time. I can't do things on the spur of the moment, I always have to be available.
>
> (Carvill 2008: 314)

> Friends are really hard. We couldn't socialise with this child needing twenty-four seven care, plus the stress. I couldn't be bothered with visitors plus they didn't understand, not having a clue.
>
> (Jones *et al.* 2003: 136)

A further result of this impact of caring is the inability to participate more broadly in the community:

> We had an active life – lots of social committees and activities – less now. Can't manage it and husband.
>
> (Ulvestad 2006: 35)

Some carers of a child with a disability describe difficulties they experience when out with their child, particularly if the child displays inappropriate behaviour:

> I feel people are looking at me thinking, ooh, she's a bad parent.
>
> (Jones *et al.* 2003: 77)

> I feel like I have to explain myself or my child, but at the same time I feel angry and think, why should I have to explain myself? I constantly feel like there's an internal battle going on.
>
> (Jones *et al.* 2003: 80)

This type of experience, in addition to the huge time commitment in caring for the child, can lead to a self-imposed isolation:

> At times it is very easy to become a recluse. It is just too hard to get out, just too hard to do this, too hard to talk about. The child tends to dominate the conversations when you're at home and when you're out.
>
> (Jones *et al.* 2003: 136)

Financial exclusion

For many carers, the caring role has significant financial implications. In the recent survey of Australian carers, their satisfaction with their ability to pay for household essentials, to afford things they would like to have, to save money, and to not worry about income covering expenses were all severely compromised in comparison with participants from the general population who completed similar surveys (Cummins *et al.* 2007). Some carers face severe time constraints and are unable to participate in paid employment. Additional costs are incurred for some carers, particularly those caring for the disabled:

> Financially it is hard on us with only one of us working, but with the needs of the children I really can't work. Anything you need for the disabled tends to be twice the price.
>
> (Fennessy *et al.* 2008: 196)

The allowance made available to carers is viewed as clearly insufficient by carers:

> We get a disability allowance for looking after them, but that works out to about thirteen cents an hour. ... So it's always going to be a financial burden, which is an awful way of looking at it, but it is.
>
> (Fennessy *et al.* 2008: 196)

Another carer of a young person with a disability indicated that dealing with the bureaucracy in order to obtain some form of financial assistance was another disempowering experience:

I wish Centrelink were easier to deal with, they are the biggest pain in the neck honestly, which is why I haven't bothered with the disability support pension. I am just not interested in dealing with government departments, they make you wait for hours and hours and feel like an idiot.

(Fennessy *et al.* 2008: 198)

Similarly, in Carvill's (2008) interviews with carers in the areas of aged care, disability and mental illness, some carers reported either reducing or relinquishing their work commitments to meet the demands of caregiving. Carers who continued to work appeared to need additional support to balance the combination of work and caring. The limitations associated with current support services were also discussed by carers. For example, if the care recipient is unwell there is no emergency support available for the care recipient which would enable the carer to go to work rather than remain with the care recipient.

Systematic exclusion

There is a substantial body of literature on the impact of caregiving, and sophisticated theories explaining the interactions between the stressors experienced by carers and their ability to manage these (Pearlin *et al.* 1990; Aneshensel *et al.* 1995; Folkman 1997). However, this knowledge appears to have had little impact on the service system, in relation to how carers are treated. Four ways of thinking about carers and their relationship with formal services have been characterised by Twigg and Atkin (1994), who have argued that how a carer is perceived by organisations and practitioners determines whether their needs are recognised and addressed. The four approaches to carers are:

1 carers as resources in which carers are seen as a means to an end of meeting the care recipient's needs;
2 carers as co-workers with whom the formal care providers work in parallel with the outcome being focused on the welfare of the care recipient;
3 carers as co-clients where the focus is on relieving the carer of strain or stress; and
4 the superseded carer in which the aim is not to support the caregiving relationship but to transcend or supersede it. (Twigg and Atkin 1994: 14–15).

Our research in the Barwon-South West region of Victoria suggests that carers are viewed as resources by most organisations and front line practitioners, but their needs are neither recognised nor addressed consistently. In fact, many support services were clear that the focus of their service was on meeting the needs of the care recipient (Carvill 2008). The following quotes from carers caring for someone with a disability typify a system that is not working cooperatively with carers:

> One of the problems is that you are dismissed as a parent, like you don't know anything. Professionals are thought to be the experts, whereas I think we are.
>
> (Fennessy *et al.* 2008: 59)

> I was told 'You're mad' when I said I wanted [care recipient] home with me. I was told I couldn't do it and a residential placement was the best option. Because he has high level needs [agency name] won't provide a service. I have had to fight to get funding and services. The system needs an overhaul.
>
> (Carvill 2008: 309)

Navigating a system that is not user-friendly is also problematic for many carers, and a disempowering experience for them:

> Everything is disjointed. If you need something that is out of the norm you have to do lots of phone calls. There's no central point. No one person to call for information.
>
> (Carvill 2008: 309)

Others commented that 'Finding services is a nightmare' (Carvill 2008: 309) and that 'I have no idea what support is available' (Carvill 2008: 309).

A number of carers interviewed indicated that there was an expectation that they would be able to specify what type of support they needed in their role, which the carers explained they could not do:

> Sometimes I get tired and feel like I need something but don't know what.
>
> (Carvill 2008: 254)

> The hardest question I was asked was by someone from [agency name]. They asked 'What do you need?' and I found this very hard to answer.
>
> (Carvill 2008: 254)

Carer self-identification of unmet support needs is problematic as such a process assumes that the carer has a detailed knowledge about the range of support services available and how the services may help to alleviate specific causes of stress. Self-identification of support needs also presumes that the carer can objectively pinpoint all sources of personal stress including both physical and emotional sources. The practitioner's failure to identify a carer's needs has important negative implications for the wellbeing of the carer. The existence of unmet needs has been found to have negative implications for the carer's wellbeing and ability to continue within the role (Gaugler *et al.* 2005).

Some interviews with carers provide further evidence of the disempowerment of the carer via the language used by professionals to describe the care recipient:

When she was newborn, she was interesting to everybody, so they kept calling her 'an interesting case', never by name, just 'an interesting case'. I said, 'She's my daughter; she's not an interesting case at all'.

(Fennessy *et al.* 2008: 211)

Health promotion implications

The negative health impact of social isolation and not being engaged or participating in one's community is acknowledged (Rosenfeld 1997; Michael *et al.* 2002). Similarly, the inability to participate in health enhancing behaviours such as physical activity is detrimental to an individual's health and wellbeing (Bauman *et al.* 2002; Teychenne *et al.* 2008). In addition, there is potentially a negative impact for both the individual and the community when volunteering activities are restricted or precluded. Volunteering is a particularly important way of being socially engaged, providing benefits to the community as a whole, to the recipients of the voluntary work, and also to the volunteers themselves. A review of the literature on volunteering suggests that people who volunteer are likely to maintain significantly higher levels of wellbeing, a strong sense of their own worth, and have better functional health than those who do not volunteer (Onyx and Warburton 2003). Importantly, there is evidence that volunteering actually improves wellbeing and functional health: it is not just that healthier people are able to volunteer (Davis *et al.* 1998; Onyx and Warburton 2003).

There are a number of systemic factors that could be altered to improve the health and wellbeing of carers. A change in the model of service provision so that carers are treated as co-clients rather than as resources, as described by Twigg and Atkin (1994), would be beneficial to carers. Such a change should result not only in more appropriate support for carers, but would also enable carers to feel that they are valued and have an important role to play as carers. They should be empowered and made to feel knowledgeable and proud rather than ignored and foolish. For carers who are in the workforce, greater flexibility in working hours and in rules for taking time off would facilitate a smoother integration of the working and caring role. Finally, more substantial financial support for carers would assist those who experience hardship and find it difficult to cope financially with the additional costs of caring.

At the community level, an enhanced awareness in general of the impact of the caring role on carers could lead to changes that would be of benefit to carers. Small gestures can at times make a substantial difference. For example, a neighbour dropping in and offering even a small amount of help, or simply having a chat with an elderly person caring for a frail aged partner could be an important social event for the carer. Within families, an increased understanding of the relationship between carer and care recipient, and of the impact of the situation on the carer, could facilitate smoother communication and perhaps some assistance from other family members. Within communities, an increased understanding of disability and mental health in general, and of the role of caregivers for people with a disability or mental health problem, may lead to a level of tolerance and support in the community that would be highly beneficial to carers and their care recipients. Roth *et al.* (2005) found that addressing carer satisfaction with the social supports available through individual and family counselling altered the stress process by changing a threatening appraisal to a more benign appraisal. This type of carer inter-vention which is aimed at enhancing the social support of spousal carers of a person with Alzheimer's disease has been found to be effective in reducing the emotional distress associated with the role.

Conclusion

The various ways in which people who provide informal care experience exclusion largely stem from the failure, at various levels, to acknowledge both the importance of, and the impact of, the role played by carers. This occurs at a systemic level and at a community or personal level. The impact of this exclusion undoubtedly contributes to poor health and wellbeing outcomes for carers. The exclusion of carers is also detrimental to the overall community, as it prevents carers from participating in their community at an optimal level.

2.7 Debating the capacity of information and communication technology to promote inclusion

Jane Maidment and Selma Macfarlane

Introduction

Discussion around the use and impact of information and communication technology (ICT) has created polarised debates about the potential of ICT to generate inclusion or exclusion. Computer mediated communication is variously heralded as a means of transcending 'sociocultural markers such as race and gender ... lead[ing] to a utopian society', and denigrated for creating 'impoverished, low-trust relationships at best and social withdrawal, at worst' (Markham 2005: 794). Similarly, it is argued that the plethora of information available via ICT can break down hierarchical access to information and power previously dependent on social position. Conversely, however, others observe that ICT has created new inequalities based on the information rich and the information poor, and one's position in controlling, or being controlled by, technological advancements. As Markham (2005) comments, such universalised and dichotomised opinions have been usefully extended to include more specific, context-based analyses, acknowledging a complex range of processes and outcomes associated with ICT in various settings. This chapter explores this diversity and some of the ways ICT has impacted on human service education, professional development, and the provision of services in specific contexts. We attempt to identify ways in which ICT may lead to social inclusion and/or exclusion for social groups with varying access to ICT.

The chapter begins with an exploration of the digital divide in the Australian context. This discussion is followed by an examination of online education, professional development and the capacity of ICT to enhance the well-being of practitioners. The chapter then focuses on the use of ICT in human services and the rise of computer mediated self help and support groups. The potential for ICT to promote and extend political participation is also explored as well as the role of ICT in global development. Throughout, the potential for inclusion and exclusion is highlighted, using examples, and critical analysis for exploring the inclusionary and exclusionary capacity of ICT.

The Australian context

The penetration of internet usage across Australia is currently estimated to be 72 per cent, indicating a 135 per cent rise since 2000 (Internet World Stats 2007). Even so there is ample evidence to indicate access to ICT delivery of information and services is extremely uneven across Australia, with factors such as location, educational status, income, ethnicity and age impacting upon access (Lloyd and Hellwig 2000). Those with poor English skills, Indigenous Australians, people over 55 and those living in remote parts of the country are less likely to use a computer at home or access the internet (Daly 2005). This 'yawning digital divide both within and across countries' has been identified in earlier global research and analysis on internet use (Guillen and Suarez 2005: 681) illustrating world wide inequity and disparity between populations who have access to the benefits of ICT and those that do not.

Enhancing telecommunications to rural and remote regions is currently a hot topic on the Australian political agenda. Individual State governments have endeavoured to resource and strengthen ICT in differing ways to promote more accessible health and educational services (State Government of Victoria, Department of Human Services 2007; Way and Webb 2007). The focus on ICT for Federal government however, has been on the development of a strategic framework to enhance the 'information economy' underpinned by an ideology of competitive tendering for the telecommunications market (Pluss 2004). There is no surprise that the push for broadband access to telecommunications coverage throughout the country coincided with Australian politicians using the internet for the first time to deliver targeted lobbying during the election year of 2007. Even so, an audit of facilities to specific Indigenous communities has concluded there are significant barriers to developing better communication systems to these populations. These barriers include poor housing and physical obstacles created by isolation, while the harsh environment makes ongoing maintenance of equipment difficult (DCITA 2002 cited in Daly 2005). Access to ICT often depends on income, education (literacy, training), race/ethnicity, age, gender, family structure, geographic location and disability; groups with the least access in Australia have been described as the rural poor, rural and urban minorities, female-headed households and young rural and urban low income households (Moffatt 1999). While the literature abounds with examples of ways in which practitioners working in rural and remote regions can use ICT to access additional professional development, it cannot be assumed that this is a universal experience.

Online education, professional development and well being of practitioners

This part of the discussion will focus on the delivery of education and professional development and support to students and practitioners located in disparate locations across the country. Particular attention will be given to identifying the enabling and inhibiting features of using differing forms of ICT for these purposes. The tensions inherent in juggling principles of social justice and equity with the pragmatic considerations of 'being seen' to deliver education and professional development will be highlighted.

Most professional bodies require practitioners to demonstrate continuing engagement with professional development activities in order to maintain accreditation and/or membership. However, for those living in rural and remote locations, potentially hundreds of kilometres away from an urban setting, accessing professional development is particularly difficult on a number of fronts. Two of the most significant inhibiters are: meeting the costs associated with travelling long distances, event registration and accommodation; and needing to employ qualified locums to provide service coverage during a worker's absence in regions where few professionally qualified personnel actually live (Taylor and Lee 2005). For practitioners in this situation the prospect of accessing professional development through ICT is appealing but not without its problems, and the cultural dimensions and implications associated with delivering education, via ICT, have remained relatively unexplored.

Even so, we know 22 per cent of the Australian population were born overseas (Australian Bureau of Statistics 2007b) while 2.5 per cent are of Aboriginal descent (Australian Bureau of Statistics 2007c). In addition recent initiatives to boost the rural and remote health workforce in Australia have seen significant numbers of qualified personnel from overseas countries being wooed to practise in these regions (ABC News Feb. 5 2008; Roach *et al.* 2007). For many within these particular cohorts English is not the first language, resulting in a disconnect, where cultural and linguistic differences are simply not taken into account in the design or delivery of online learning. While professional development and higher education endeavours in this country continue to be delivered exclusively in English, an immediate cultural barrier exists for some in accessing these resources, in terms of having compromised speed in reading, writing and constructing ideas in English, mostly without the benefit of visual cues (Dillon *et al.* 2007: 156).

The dominance of English in virtual education contributes also to an ongoing marginalisation of local indigenous languages (Goodfellow *et al.* 2001). We note that the impact of ICT in terms of compromising cultural diversity is rarely addressed in the professional development or higher education literature.

These problems need to be weighed up against the obvious benefits reported by practitioners in using ICT to overcome the isolation experienced while working in rural and remote locations. There is ample evidence of the growing use of email, instant messaging, teleconferencing and videoconferencing for peer support and supervision by a range of disciplines (Russel and Perris 2003), resulting in significant savings in travel costs and professional time without compromising on quality of the supervision (McCarty and Clancy 2002). Recent research amongst Australian occupational therapists found that while practitioners in geographically isolated areas have less ready access to

computer hardware than urban colleagues, levels of confidence and familiarity with using a range of ICT for professional consultation and education
were highest amongst rural practitioners (Taylor and Lee 2005). These findings reflect those of earlier studies that note the rapid uptake of ICT in isolated regions where practitioners are more reliant upon these modes of
communication for connecting with others to access professional advice and
support (Australian New Zealand Telehealth Committee 2000). Meanwhile,
practitioners in regional and urban locations are more likely to encounter
colleagues in person at meetings, case conferences, and in-service education
gatherings, and as such have less need for getting 'online' or video conferencing.

The blurring of domestic and professional worlds is a further confounding
feature in analysing the inclusive and exclusive dimensions of ICT. While 24/7
accessibility (for some) is one of the frequently cited benefits of ICT, this level
of connectedness generates an expectation that practitioners and educators
will attend to work matters in times that have traditionally been considered
'out of work hours', being available to work around the clock (Wynhausen
2008). In this respect elements of changing industrial relations, increased
consumer expectations and ICT usage intersect, demonstrating that economic,
political, social and educational dimensions associated with ICT accessibility
cannot be separated out. Within a climate of strident economic rationalism,
practitioners and educators come under increasing pressure to attend to client
matters and professional development needs during evenings and weekends.
Paradoxically the seemingly empowering features of accessible ICT can
quickly become disempowering and particularly problematic in a climate of
the global market economy.

For better or worse, the workplaces of first world human service practitioners have indeed been revolutionised by developments in ICT, as we
explore in the following section.

Human service databases: promoting social inclusion through developments in ICT?

As human service/welfare organisations have grown, along with client numbers, the use of computer-based record keeping promised greater simplicity,
storage capacity, uniformity and efficiency for workers, making it easier to
calculate workloads and throughput, and generate statistics on client populations and service effectiveness. From social security to child protection, it is
hard to imagine how large client caseloads could be managed today without
the use of ICT. So how has the new 'techno-habitat' (Dyer-Witheford 1999,
cited in Garrett 2005: 530) of social and welfare workers impacted on practice,
and on promoting a more socially inclusive and just society?

Databases are capable of generating large amounts of statistical information, which allows organisations to track large numbers of clients through
their system, provide details necessary to lobby for and maintain funding,
provide indicators around the occurrence and nature of social problems, and

inform program planning to meet the needs of client groups (Donovan and Jackson 1991; Thorpe 1994). These enhanced capacities can potentially increase the capability of organisations to understand better and meet the needs of service users, promoting social inclusion through targeted (re)distribution of resources. At the same time, it is argued that if workers become overly reliant on computer-generated statistics, categories and procedures, professional knowledge and experience is devalued, with a number of negative outcomes. There are concerns that databases in large bureaucracies may mask the complexities of human experience, take time away from direct work with clients, enable the mis-use of client information, and problematically lump individuals into categories that obviate diversity within social groupings (Ahmad and Sheldon 1993; Thorpe 1994; Garrett 2005). Reducing complex human experiences to quick and easy individualised 'solutions' can minimise wider structural issues; this is worrying if inclusion is to be based on respect for diversity and acknowledgment of structural inequality (Garrett 2005). Australian social work academic Philip Mendes highlights that social inclusion is about process as well as outcome. He stresses the importance of developing processes that seek to include rather than to exclude, and that reflect a valuing of and respect for all members of a community even if they hold conflicting views (2008: 99–100). This definition extends notions of social inclusion that focus only on outcomes: access to resources and participation in mainstream society.

Client databases allow for greater ease in accessing and sharing large amounts of information (Garrett 2005). Garrett uses the evocative term 'digital shadows' to describe the ways in which 'data selves' are created as indicators of a family's or individual's worth and deservedness, potentially eroding the civil liberties of users – or potential users – of child welfare services, in an attempt to create social order, within human services themselves, and more widely. Peterson (1994) critiques the role of technology in the surveillance and discipline functions of welfare organisations, which, he argues, may lead workers to objectify service recipients, rather than participate in more dialogic forms of engagement.

The wider socio-political context in which ICT has burgeoned is significant to a critical analysis. Advances in the use of ICT in human services have been accompanied by tighter targeting of welfare and human services aligned with neo-liberal/conservative discourse around the wastefulness of the welfare state. In such an environment, the focus is on individualised deviance or deficit, and the assessment of risks posed by individuals to the 'good society' is foregrounded. Bessant (2003) discusses the dominance of risk-based thinking in Australian social policy and human service agencies and the rise of computerised 'risk instruments' such as the Job Seekers Classification Index (JSCI) in the management of unemployed clients (see, for example, McDonald *et al.* 2003). Bessant critiques the technical rationality purportedly afforded by such instruments, suggesting that risk-informed practice is often excessively oriented to control and domination, which minimises professional judgement and compromises the creation of respectful and trusting relationships (2003: 32). According to McDonald *et al.* (2003: 520), 'The JSCI is a technology that reduces multiple interview responses into a single number and barriers to employment into multiple sites of psychological intervention, thus further transposing the problem of unemployment into the field of scientific knowledge and therapeutic rectification.' This not only categorises the person in relation to their level of risk of remaining unemployed but also ignores the structural issues that may have led to the person's exclusion from meaningful and empowered participation in the labour market. A form of social inclusion is generated that is top-down, authoritarian and simplistic, enabling the state to 'police the socially marginalised', based on a 'narrow, normative and prescriptive view of the world and economic relationships' (Garrett 2005: 543).

While the preceding discussion has raised some questions as to the emancipatory nature of ICT in particular contexts, the next section paints a more optimistic picture of ways in which ICT may open doors to knowledge sharing and enhanced accessibility of human services.

The use of ICT to enhance direct service provision

Some forms of ICT have undoubtedly expanded the parameters of direct service delivery for health and human services. For example, telephone and online counselling has burgeoned and appears to have provided emancipatory possibilities to many seeking confidential and easily accessible help and assistance to the ICT literate. Australians are familiar with a national service to children and young people called the Kids Help Line – a free 24-hour telephone and online counselling service aimed at helping young people to 'manage their own lives more effectively' (Reid and Caswell 2005: 269). According to Reid and Caswell (2005: 272), over 400 young people accessed the service via email weekly, and more than 250 made contact via real-time web counselling. Online service users were mostly girls aged between 15 and 18 years, while boys were more likely to use the telephone component of the service. Despite little advertising, growth in demand for online counselling rose annually by over forty per cent since 1999, indicating that the service fulfils a needed role, with the most common issue raised both on the telephone and online being that of family relationships. Reid and Caswell (2005) conclude that the success of the service stems from its ease of use, particularly as many young people are familiar with computers and online techniques, ease of access as compared to physically attending a counselling session, control over time of access, and confidentiality. It is also a service available to people who are geographically isolated.

ICT has also created new avenues for isolated professionals to connect with the expertise of others. Telehealth practices allow client care to be conducted across distance, using a range of technologies, to conduct virtual visits, videoconference, and email information and advice. In Australia, Harrison and Lee (2006) observed that e-health provided health information to professionals and consumers via more than 100,000 websites, aimed at increased efficiency in health care, improved quality of care, and empowerment of patients/consumers (Harrison and Lee 2006). Internet sites provide almost limitless sources of health information (as compared to a brief visit with a practitioner); however, the sheer amount of information available from a variety of sources may make obtaining credible, accurate information difficult.

For human service workers across a wide spectrum of practice, ICT access can allow for easy communication with other social/welfare workers and agencies via emails, electronic circulation of documents and information sharing. The internet, as well as increasing numbers of e-journals and e-databases, allows workers to extend their knowledge around specific fields of practice, social policy, and social issues, by accessing professional mega-sites, organisational websites, policy information and knowledge relevant to specific fields of practice. Workers in isolated roles have the potential to connect with others via, for example, participation in internet discussion groups. These are all practices that enable access to resources at an almost unprecedented level, at least for those who are suitably resourced.

Access and activism

The capacity of ICT to engender social relationships and support – virtual communities – has been discussed by many authors. From rural jobseekers (McQuaid *et al.* 2004) to remote area youth (Notley and Tacchi 2005), to public housing tenants (Hopkins *et al.* 2004), to institutionalised elders (Mickus and Luz 2001), and transnational migrants (Panagakos and Horst 2006), it is suggested that ICT can fill a role in connecting people in supportive, enabling or sustaining ways. But do these virtual communities actually enhance social inclusion, and if so, how?

One example that explores the capacity for ICT to promote social inclusion is related to transnational migration, a potentially isolating experience. Panagakos and Horst (2006) examined how the social worlds and networks of transnational migrants were mediated through ICT. Specifically, they explored how cheap long distance telephony, mobile phones and text messaging, the internet, emails, blogging and chat rooms were incorporated into the daily lives of transnational populations to maintain links with their previous homeland or with other new settlement areas. They observed that engagement with and access to 'diasporic media' (Karim 2003, cited in Panagakos and Horst 2006: 111) depended on location (variable infrastructure), gender (with women sometimes unable to access technology) and status. While concerns about surveillance and an over-reliance on online groups were identified in their case studies, the capacity of ICT to provide an alternative to mainstream media and communication channels was considered advantageous (Panagakos and Horst 2006). What this means in terms of social inclusion is of interest: social inclusion is often defined as social and financial inclusion in *mainstream* economic and political systems and opportunities (Mendes 2008: 167).

However, at times ICT may enable sub-cultures to build their own strong networks rather than assimilate to mainstream norms and systems. This raises important questions as to ways in which dominant versions of 'social inclusion' may be more about assimilation into dominant norms and values than self determination. As Spandler (2007: 12) puts it, 'The demand for social inclusion is paradoxical in that it both expresses a genuine desire to tackle the consequences of social inequality and yet at the same time could become co-opted as a modern form of moral and social governance which reproduces and legitimises the prevailing socio-economic order.' We next explore some of the ways groups use ICT to resist co-option and construct alternative discourses: creating, perhaps, social inclusion on their own terms.

The internet has been lauded for its potential to create 'virtual public spheres for democratic dialogue' and information sharing (Jensen 2003: 29). Chen *et al.* (2006: 2) specify four core areas of electronic democracy: political equality, popular control of government, civil liberties and human rights, and quality of public debate. They suggest that ICT today provides new and unparalleled possibilities for many people to 'participate in interactive content, and be a simultaneous producer and consumer of content' (Chen *et al.* 2006: 5). Further, they observe, 'if information is power, then the internet clearly can act as a democratising and equalising force … [and] a forum to those who might previously have been unable or unwilling to engage in debate on issues of concern to them' (Chen *et al.* 2006: 8). So, how does ICT, and particularly the internet, create pathways for liberatory political engagement, information sharing and empowered dialogue?

In Australia, political action does indeed take place on the internet, with e-groups such as Moveon.org., Getup.org.au and Indy Media increasingly mobilising political involvement. Getup uses new technology 'to empower Australians to have their say on important national issues' and boasted over 230,000 subscribers in 2007 (Getup 2007). During the 2007 federal election, Getup's election blog provided a discussion forum, as well as a 'make your vote count' interactive questionnaire matching political/policy sentiments with the most resonant party. Using ICT, political lobbying and organising can evolve across time and space. Information can be shared via websites and newsgroups, for example in support of asylum seekers (see Meikle 2004 – 'We are all boat people campaign') and other social concerns. When the Howard federal government launched its controversial Crisis Intervention measures into Indigenous communities in the Northern Territory, grassroots organisations such as Women for Wik monitored the intervention and distributed weekly emails to subscribers across the country, providing links, media releases and updates on the intervention.

Activist social justice and advocacy groups appear to be using ICT to resist exclusionary and oppressive aspects of globalisation, such as the expansion of global capitalism, the exploitation of weaker states by multinational corporations and the erosion of indigenous cultures and environments. They demand inclusion in political dialogue based on their own interpretations of social reality and alternative visions for the present and future. McNutt and Menon (2008) suggest that 'cyberactivism' may be vital to the future of advocacy in human services, particularly in the current neo-liberal environment, which has created tough times for social welfare advocates. The internet, they observe, provides a new arena for global activism, allowing activists to 'organise more supporters with fewer resources over greater distances' and develop and share information (McNutt and Menon 2008: 33–34).

These examples suggest that ICT may indeed be capable of fostering and enabling dialogue and emancipatory projects in revolutionary ways. Srinivasan (2006) proposes that ICT has the potential to remove 'the dichotomies of "oppressor-oppressed" [and] to allow a constructive dialogue wherein shared visions and aspirations emerge' (355): a participatory and power sharing form of social inclusion. Srinivasan distinguishes between emancipatory community based ICT development, and that which leaves oppressive and unequal power structures intact or exacerbated. He critically questions assumptions around development and information access that do not acknowledge or ask who or what is driving the agenda. The imposition of dominant (Western) paradigms, he observes, can create dependency on the providers of technology and impose culturally imperialist agendas, including the type of information to be accessed and for what purpose. The antidote to this top down and oppressive approach is to adopt a process reliant on community input, local context and knowledge, and cultural appropriateness. Srinivasan (2006) describes the 'Village Incubator project' in which community processes and goals emerged over a period of reflection, facilitated by NGOs and ICT experts who provided video and other visual technologies but did not dictate how they were to be used. Through a process of community meetings and media created by community members, communities were engaged in a way that recognised development as a shared process aimed at uncovering deeper Indigenous wisdom and community directed vision (Friere 1968, cited in Srinivasan 2006).

Similarly, Puri and Sahay (2003) observe the failure of ICT projects that inferiorise Indigenous knowledge and leave oppressive power relationships intact. They refer to Habermas's ideal speech situation as a way of addressing 'this problem of knowledge integration' (183); ICT users, they say, must be actively involved in defining the agenda of development in the local context and how ICT is used to meet community defined goals. Indeed, this may provide a model or framework for critical analysis of specific and contextualised uses of ICT and its inclusionary and exclusionary capacities. The 'ideal speech situation' is a form of inclusionary communication based on equality of access and equality of participation in dialogue amongst interest groups (Habermas 1987).

Conclusion

Given the diverse implications of various forms and uses of ICT in specific contexts, polarised debates constructing ICT in fixed categories of 'emancipatory' or 'oppressive' (or inclusionary or exclusionary) seem fraught. Critical frameworks are crucial in examining the use and impact of ICT locally and globally. It is unlikely that the use of ICT will abate in the near future: those concerned with social justice and equality will need to engage critically in assessing its impact and inclusionary potential in specific contexts. Jacques Ellul's '76 Reasonable Questions to Ask About any Technology' also provides an interesting framework for critical reflection on the emancipatory or oppressive effects of ICT. Ellul's questions ask us to consider the ecological, social, practical, moral, ethical, vocational, metaphysical, political and aesthetic value of any technology, including questions such as

> What are its effects on the health of the planet and of the person? Does it preserve or reduce cultural diversity? Does it empower community members? Who does it benefit? Can it be repaired (by an ordinary person)? What is lost in using it? To what extent does it distance agent from effect? Does it concentrate or equalise power?

Such questions might help us understand the inclusionary and exclusionary capacities of ICT in specific contexts as we engage with the world at local and global levels.

2.8 The Reading Discovery program: increasing social inclusion of marginalised families

Karen Stagnitti and Claire Jennings

Creating a socially inclusive society requires the removal of barriers and the investment in action to bring about conditions where all children and adults participate as valued, respected, and contributing members of society. In this chapter we show changes in families' social inclusion which resulted from a program designed to increase the preliterate skills of children by building parents' awareness and confidence.

When young people are socially included they feel valued and supported and acquire a social capital of their own (Holland *et al.* 2007). Social capital is both 'bonding' capital (that is, family relationships and networks of trust) and 'bridging' capital (outwards looking social networks) (Holland *et al.* 2007). Both types of social capital are considered important to social inclusion and an imbalance can lead to restricted social inclusion of the individual through negative social contact within networks (Holland *et al.* 2007; Stafford *et al.* 2003) and negative social environments (Wen *et al.* 2005).

Social inclusion during childhood is especially important since children are dependent on the quality of their family, community and school environment for positive mental health and wellbeing. Social exclusion, once established, tracks across the lifecourse. Those who enter school in a vulnerable state will tend to be less healthy, experience lower levels of wellbeing and be more likely to end up in socially marginalised positions as life unfolds (Hertzman 2002).

Marginalised families

In 2004, a review in the UK of the impact of government policy on social inclusion of children identified nine areas associated with a risk of social exclusion (Buchanan 2007); seven of these are associated with living in disadvantage and being marginalised such as intergenerational poverty, low income, low socioeconomic status and socioeconomic disadvantage. Socioeconomic disadvantage has negative effects on the development of children in relation to cognitive, emotional and social wellbeing and development (Attree 2004; Evans 2004; Huebner 2000; McLoyd 1998). Children living in disadvantage are more likely to receive limited health care services, live in single parent families and drop out of school (Pressey and Holm 2006). The child's home environment is typified by inadequate play materials and books, lack of, or unsafe, play spaces; exposure to less responsive parenting, limited parental encouragement, stimulation and assistance (Attree 2004; Cooper 2000; Evans 2004).

Insensitive, rejecting and unresponsive parenting during the early years results in an insecure attachment relationship between the caregiver and child (Aber and Allen 1987; Egeland and Sroufe 1981). When parents are not responsive or do not interact verbally in an extensive way with their children they are not modelling speech where children learn the nuances of language or the syntax of progressively more complex sentences and vocabulary, thus limiting the child's language experience and development (Allen and Oliver 1982; McLoyd 1998). Marginalised families have fewer resources which preclude their children from gaining rich and varied life experiences. This impacts on reading-readiness as all readers rely on their prior knowledge when making sense of text and in predicting what comes next in a sentence or a story. Children from these environments lack school readiness. For healthy development, children require supportive environments that provide enriching play experiences with materials such as props, books and toys (Allessandri 1991; Allen and Oliver 1982).

Vocabulary generation in the preschool years can realise up to 14,000 words, the outcome of healthy and varied interactions between the mother or caregiver and the child (Wells 1985a, 1985b, 1987). If the main care-giver is ill or preoccupied by adverse life circumstances then the child is at risk of language delay of up to two years behind their peers. This lag in learning readiness affects performance in the first year of school which further disadvantages the child in learning potential and is associated with social exclusion.

In Australia, Makin and Diaz noted the effects on literacy development when children were from marginalised families:

> certain groups of children appear to be less likely to meet government benchmarks in literacy. Children who are Indigenous, from low income homes, with limited access to print materials in their homes ... , who speak languages other than English, and, increasingly, who are male, are less likely to reach the benchmarks (2004: 74).

Figures from the National School English Literacy Survey in Australia (Australian Council for Educational Research 1997) demonstrated that 27 per cent of children were not meeting the reading standard. This percentage increased to 38 per cent for children with low socioeconomic backgrounds and 81 per cent for children with an Indigenous background. Long term studies of early intervention programs such as the High/Scope Perri Pre School Program in the United States (Schweinhart *et al.* 1993) have documented significant improvements in literacy and social skills, as well as the cost effectiveness of providing appropriate support to young children and families in the early years of life (Smedley and Syme 2001).

Literacy as a pathway to social connectedness

Children who are exposed to early literacy activities (e.g. nursery rhymes, repetitive and cumulative stories) are more likely to adapt to formal literacy classes at school and have amongst the highest comprehension levels by age eight (Goswami and East 2000). Children whose parents read to them become better readers and perform better at school (Snow *et al.* 1999). Parents' impact on their child's development is significant and the quality of parental stimulation plays an important role in either supporting or hindering child development (McCain and Mustard 1999). Healthy attachment, trust and security, curiosity, a sense of humour and empathy can be fostered through parents' daily reading of books to children, particularly when parents are aware of which books to choose, and respond to and interact with the text and illustrations to foster emergent literacy skills in the developing child. Although it is recognised that the impact of reading programs may extend beyond language and literacy skills, the impact of reading programs on the social health and wellbeing of parents and children has rarely been examined (Nelson *et al.* 2005).

Research focused on beginning reading skills has shown that these interventions may improve a child's social functioning in the classroom (Nelson *et al.* 2005). A study that explored social inclusion in marginalised families in a rural community by addressing the pre-literacy skills of children through parent involvement is the Reading Discovery program described in this chapter. This research produced baseline data on the social networks and social support of marginalised families and a description of the social networks of marginalised families after involvement in the program.

Reading Discovery program

Reading Discovery is a family literacy program aimed at parents and their preschool children in marginalised rural groups. The program was developed by Claire Jennings, who has expertise in literacy and early education (Masters Education and Arts) and who is the program manager. Reading Discovery is based on research around the social nature of knowledge and language acquisition and how children learn language and their consequent learning and literacy development (Vygotsky 1997). Many of the critical periods for brain development are over by the age of six, with the most vital stage in children's development being in the first three years (McCain and Mustard 2002). Hence, Reading Discovery targets children from birth and their families. The program is founded on establishing relationships with parents who work as partners in the program to maximise skills growth in their children. Parents of children aged 0–5 years are educated about the vital role they play in the reading readiness of their children by school age. This partnership supports ongoing learning at home as well as strengthening family bonds in the early years of a child's life. Reading Discovery takes a whole of community approach (see

Figure 2.1) where marginalised families work beside staff on a one-on-one basis (centre of the circle) and then families are assisted and encouraged to integrate with the community in activities such as play groups, libraries and community systems including Family Day Care, kindergartens and schools.

Reading Discovery is delivered through Community Connections, a not-for-profit non-government agency in Victoria, Australia. Families are referred from the Family Service Programs within Community Connections and after referral the Reading Discovery program manager or a qualified practitioner meets the family in their home and introduces the program. Weekly home visits by practitioners or specially trained volunteers model the strategies of

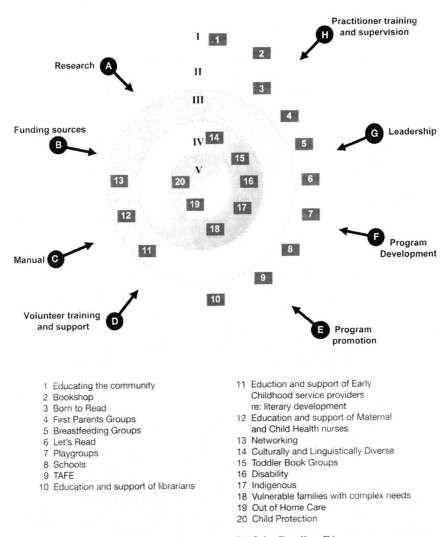

1 Educating the community
2 Bookshop
3 Born to Read
4 First Parents Groups
5 Breastfeeding Groups
6 Let's Read
7 Playgroups
8 Schools
9 TAFE
10 Education and support of librarians

11 Eduction and support of Early Childhood service providers re: literary development
12 Education and support of Maternal and Child Health nurses
13 Networking
14 Culturally and Linguistically Diverse
15 Toddler Book Groups
16 Disability
17 Indigenous
18 Vulnerable families with complex needs
19 Out of Home Care
20 Child Protection

Figure 2.1 The whole of community approach of the Reading Discovery program

reading to, playing with, and dialogistic interaction with children. Through the program children are exposed to rich language interaction at a crucial time in their cognitive, social and emotional development.

Reading Discovery recognises that children in vulnerable families may have significant language deprivation which will restrict their future learning potential and social inclusion. Whilst Reading Discovery respects the cultural capital of families in the lower socioeconomic sector, children in such families may be disadvantaged linguistically and cognitively in wider social settings such as kindergarten and school. The focus on language stimulation through chanting nursery rhymes and reading and discussing fiction (and non-fiction) with preschoolers is an attempt to address this imbalance and is supported by studies which demonstrate that the early experience of stories is the single best preparation for school (Wells 1985a, 1985b, 1987). Wells found that listening to stories being read was positively correlated with measures of knowledge of literacy taken on school entry and reading comprehension taken at age seven.

Reading Discovery also incorporates playing out the story with the practitioners and volunteers modelling to parents how to engage with children in play. In marginalised families, it is common to find that parents were not adequately parented themselves. Thus Reading Discovery is structured around strategies to increase parent/child bonding including shared reading, interacting with the read-aloud process, and imaginative story-play. Through these strategies, parents spend quality time with their children. Playing out the stories that children have seen and/or heard reinforces the understanding of the story and studies have shown that acting out the story through play increases story comprehension, understanding of story structure and understanding of narrative (Christie 1994; Pellegrini and Galda 1993). Nicoloupoulou (2005) suggested that playing and narrative (storytelling) are the opposite ends of a continuum with playing being the acting out of the story and the storytelling being the verbal expression of story. Nevertheless, they are related so when one is interrupted, so is the other. Since most reading material for beginning readers is narrative, the understanding of story structure in the preschool years helps children to think sequentially and predict what type of words will come next in a sentence, demonstrating implicit understandings of narrative text structures.

The study

A six-month evaluation of the Reading Discovery program was carried out to:

1 measure any changes that occurred in children's language, social and pretend play development;
2 gauge any changes in the parent's understanding of literacy and the home literacy environment;
3 track any changes in social inclusion of the families.

Aims one and two have been reported elsewhere (Jennings and Stagnitti 2007, Stagnitti and Jennings 2007). This chapter is concerned with Aim three of the study.

Instrument

To map the social inclusion of families, an eco map of social networks with levels of social support (see Figure 2.2) was used to measure social inclusion. There was an eco-map for each parent/carer and each child in the family. On the eco-map there were four quadrants with the quadrants representing (in a clockwise direction) social connections with family, health and welfare professionals, peers within the health/welfare system, and peers and adults outside the health/welfare system. There were three concentric circles that made up the eco-map. The inner circle represented close and strong social connections and those further out in the circles represented weaker social relationships.

Procedure

Before the research began, ethical approval was gained. A quasi-experimental design was used where families in the Reading Discovery program (one group) were pre and post tested. Families were recruited through Community Connections and were informed of the study by the Reading Discovery Project

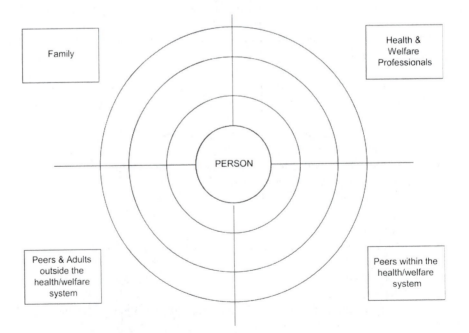

Figure 2.2 The eco-map used in data collecting

manager. If the family consented to be in the study, a time was arranged when a home visit could be made to gather the data. Parents who were literate were asked to fill in the eco-map. For parents who were not literate, the worker interviewed the parent working through the quadrants on the eco-map. The workers who assessed the families were not the volunteers who carried out the Reading Discovery program.

After the initial assessment, the families undertook the Reading Discovery program for six months. Families had weekly home visits (excluding school holidays), initially with the project manager followed by trained volunteers. During these one hour home visits children were exposed to stimulating language and social interactions. The weekly visits involved discussions with parents about selection of quality books for their children that were developmentally appropriate and how parents could foster language development and reading readiness for school. The volunteers also modelled for parents reading and imaginative story-play related to what had been read to and dialogued with the children.

Volunteers who carried out the program were recruited by Community Connections after they had been interviewed by the Program Manager and staff from the Family Services Team. Volunteers needed to demonstrate a background in either education or librarianship, or have had experience in the area of early childhood. Before the study began, volunteers completed a compulsory training package in two parts. Part 1 of the training package was a three hour training package across the Agency's services. Part 2 of the training was the completion of a day's training in the Reading Discovery program. The training program covered language and literacy development in the preschool years; the developmental stages from birth to age six years; criteria for selection of appropriate books and rhymes; keeping of client records; and key factors needed for life-long learning, for example, listening skills, concentration and curiosity. Volunteers also undertook another half day training on how pretend play relates to literacy acquisition. Volunteers were monitored at six-weekly or bi-monthly meetings with each family's case manager as well as meetings with the Reading Discovery Program Manager.

The parents were surveyed again after six months' involvement in the program. A time was organised for workers to visit families to complete the eco-map. For the follow up, the workers who undertook the assessments were again not involved in the delivery of the Reading Discovery program and therefore impartial.

Participants

Parent participants and family characteristics

Twenty families consented to be in the study; however only 19 families completed all the surveys. In 18 families, the female adult filled out the surveys and in two families the adult male filled out the surveys. The age of the parents (including Foster Carers) ranged from 17 years to 61 years. The mean age of the parents was 33.3 years with a standard deviation of 12 years, that is, most parents were aged between 21 and 45 years. In 17 of the families, the parents were the biological parents of the child, and in three families foster parents cared for the children. Nine family units included a married couple and in five family units the couple were living in a de-facto relationship. In four of the families the parents had been separated and in two families other relationships comprised the family, such as grandparents looking after the children. In five families there was a parent of Australian Aboriginal or Torres Strait Islander descent. In two of the families, the parents were born overseas (Sudanese). The number of children in the families ranged from one to five with three children being the average number of children per family. The families presented with a range of issues including: children in protective care; parents experiencing mental health issues or drug and alcohol addiction; parents with poor education; single parents; Indigenous and immigrant status families.

Seven of the parent participants (either mother or father carer) were employed full time and five were employed part time. Thirteen of the families had an annual income of less than $42,000 per year. Twelve of the 19 families indicated that they could not raise $2,000 in a week for an emergency. Five of the 19 mothers (26 per cent) had completed high school and the majority of mothers had some high school education (47 per cent). Two mothers had gone to a vocational college. Eight of the 19 fathers had some high school (42 per cent) and a further four had completed high school (21 per cent). One father had a university degree. Seventeen families spoke English only and two families spoke Arabic.

Children participants

In the initial assessment there were 24 children in the sample. On the follow up assessment after six months, data on children from 11 families were obtained. Of the 11 children on follow up, data from eight children could be paired. At the beginning of the study the mean age of these eight children was 44 months with the age range being from 22 months to 61 months. There were six girls and two boys in this sample.

Results

Nineteen families of the 20 families filled in the eco-map before the program and 11 families completed the eco-map after six months' involvement in the program. Of these 11 families, eight family sets of data for mother (that is, the female carer), father (that is, the male carer) and child were able to be matched. If a family had filled in more than one eco-map for a child, the data were collated into one set of data for children in the family. Data are reported here for the matched data set only. The loss of families from the study was due to some families moving from the region or children taken into protective care. Such circumstances are common in the demographic of the sample.

Social connections in the matched data set

Eight sets of matched data were available. To analyse any changes in social connections over the six month period, Woolcock's (1998) method of analysis of social capital was used. Woolcock's model includes social networks and social support within two types of social capital: 'bridging' capital (weak relations with numerous people) and 'bonding' capital (strong ties with a small group of people). Bridging capital is important for access to resources in society that are beyond a person's immediate circle. Bridging capital assists a person to be autonomous within society because that person has access to many resources. Bonding capital is important on a day to day level as connections are stronger and more intimate and bonding capital embeds a person within a group. Together these two types of social connections make up informal and formal social networks. Informal networks are looser, more individual connections while formal networks include organised groups. Woolcock's analysis recognises informal and formal networks in both bridging capital (called autonomy in Woolcock's analysis) and bonding capital (called embeddedness in Woolcock's analysis). The assumption of Woolcock's model is that there needs to be a balance of elements within the four quadrants of informal and formal networks across bridging and bonding capital. For example, social relationships that embed people to the exclusion of allowing them wider connections in society can be damaging.

Table 2.1 summarises the changes for each of the eight families within Woolcock's analytical framework. For mother carers, there was a reported increase in their social autonomy across both informal and formal networks as well as increased embeddedness in formal networks. For father carers, there was a reported increase in social connections in the macro level in both autonomy and embeddedness. The child data showed increased social connections (as reported by carers) in macro embeddedness (i.e. involvement in more formal social groups) and in the micro autonomy quadrant (looser networks on an informal basis). Reading Discovery program staff were reported by families to have become important in their lives with families listing Reading Discovery at Level 1 or Level 2 across both health professionals and peers within the health system.

Further analysis of the data revealed that not all cells in the eco-map were filled in by all families. The straightforward interpretation of this is that it indicates no social connections for these levels or areas. Furthermore, for three of the families, there were some areas of the eco-map filled in by the mother before the Reading Discovery Program that were left empty on the eco-map filled in after the Program. It is not known if this is because these relationships were assumed by the participants and they noted only strengthening relationships with a wider circle of people, or if family relationships really had lessened, or if they did not feel like filling in the eco-map in detail.

Table 2.1 Changes for families after 6 months of Reading Discovery Program

Family	Autonomy		Embeddedness	
	Micro	Macro	Micro	Macro
Family 1				
Mother		More services	Friends	Sudanese community
Father		More services		
Child	Library story time Childcare			
Family 2				
Mother	Distant friends	More services	Extended family	
Child	Kindergarden and day care	More services	Extended family	
Family 3				
Mother		More services		
Father	Work friends	More services		
Child		More services		
Family 4				
Mother/ Father				Dancing class Kidex group Support group for carers
Child				Dancing class Kidex group
Family 5				
Mother/ Father				Support group
Child		More services		
Family 6				
Mother		More services	Friends	English class
Father		More services		Sudanese Community
Child				Swimming classes

Table 2.1 *(continued)*

Family	Autonomy		Embeddedness	
	Micro	Macro	Micro	Macro
Family 7	No change reported			
Family 8				
Mother	Neighbours Work colleagues	More services	Friends	

Note: As data on the eco-mapping was collected under family, peers without and within the health system and health system professionals, the grid below explains how the eco-map data was categorised according to Woolcock

	Micro	Macro
autonomy	Informal, loose wider relationships e.g., kinder, day care, more distant friends	Formal, loose wider relationships. That is health services for this data
embeddedness	Informal bonding relationships e.g., family relationships and peers outside health system	Formal bonding relationships such as associations, classes and groups

Accounting for other changes that may have occurred

As the research design used in this study did not have a comparison group (that is, there was no group of families who did not undertake the Reading Discovery program but who shared similar characteristics), further analysis was undertaken to ascertain if there were any other changes in the families' lives that may have contributed to the results. Results were analysed for employment status, income and housing. There was no significant change in the employment status of the carers, household income, the adequacy of housing or type of housing before and after the program.

Five families moved from the area during the study and this accounted for the reduced availability of these families for follow up. No data are available for these families. Of the six families remaining where matched sets of eco-map data were not available before and after the program, the data that were available on family demographics indicated that the families' employment and income situation had not altered over the six months of the program.

Discussion: social inclusion of families

Family and community networks were particularly important for Indigenous and Sudanese families. Similar findings were reported by Holland *et al.* (2007) for Caribbean families. After involvement in the Reading Discovery program mother carers reported increases in their social inclusion in informal and formal networks outside their intimate networks, that is, in their social autonomy. They also increased their formal networks that embedded them within their communities. Children were also reported to have increased their peer relationships (both informal and formal) and were receiving more services within the health services sector (e.g. occupational therapist and paediatrician). As Pressey and Holm (2006) had noted that children living in poverty were more likely to receive limited health care services, this result demonstrates that children from disadvantaged families can increase their access to health services when included in an early education intervention program. Father carers indicated an increase in looser formal social networks.

The data reported in this study are self-report data by the participants. It is their perception of what is important to them in terms of social inclusion. The families in this study displayed a range of social connections across all areas of Woolcock's (1998) framework. After the program, greater autonomy in social connections of the families, particularly the mother carers, was shown. It cannot be said that involvement in the Reading Discovery program caused this increase. It can only be said that the Reading Discovery program was regarded as important by the families involved, with mother carers listing Reading Discovery as important to them more than the fathers.

Social inclusion data in this study focused on health professionals and peers within the health system as well as family and peers outside the health system. As health professionals deliver services, they become part of families' macro autonomy level of social interaction. For some families, health professionals became peers within the health system. Health professionals are within the sphere of giving access to resources outside the families' immediate social circle. Families' increased skills in literacy enable and empower them to become more autonomous in their social interactions, allowing them to engage in a wide range of social connections. This is a community aim of Reading Discovery (see Figure 2.1) and this aim was achieved, particularly with mother carers and with the children as there was an increase in families' involvement with playgroups, parent groups and the local library.

There is very little literature on literacy programs and social connectedness. This small study is a step towards understanding changes in families' social connections leading to greater social inclusion within their communities. The Reading Discovery program is specifically designed to work beside children and their carers/parents from families who are seen as marginalised. Social inclusion through wider social networks and social supports were increased after involvement in the program. Working with parents and showing them their important role in the literacy development of their children is an investment in action to increase children's developmental skills in language, social skills and play ability (Jennings and Stagnitti 2007; Stagnitti and Jennings 2007) so that the effects of marginalisation, particularly for the mothers and children of these families, is reduced and social inclusion increased.

2.9 Immigration and social exclusion: examining health inequalities of immigrants through acculturation lenses

Andre M.N. Renzaho

Introduction

Over the last three decades, the number of people migrating from developing to developed countries has been increasing in stepwise fashion as a result of insecurity, war and poverty. Such mass population movement has resulted in dramatic demographic transformations of most developed countries (Organisation for Economic Co-operation and Development 2007). The latest demographic data indicate that about 4 million new immigrants entered OECD countries on a permanent basis in 2005, an increase of 10 per cent from 2004 (Organisation for Economic Co-operation and Development 2007). In Australia, the 2006 census data indicate that more than one in five Australians (22.2 per cent) were born overseas, a pattern that has remained constant since 1996. The overseas-born population increased in number between 1996 and 2006 by 13 per cent, from around 3.9 million to 4.4 million (Australian Bureau of Statistics 2007d). Although a considerable proportion of Australian residents born overseas (including refugees and humanitarian entrants) come from countries recently affected by war and political unrest (Australian Bureau of Statistics 2007d), at a global level, migration for family reunion is the dominant reason for the inflows, and labour immigration is expanding, while humanitarian migration (including refugees and asylum seekers) has been declining (Organisation for Economic Co-operation and Development 2007).

Regardless of their migration status, cultural differences and different expectations characterise new settlers in Australia and other OECD countries. New entrants experience varying inequalities ranging from difficulties establishing social networks, finding accommodation or employment, learning English, and looking after their general health. However, the level of inequality differs according to the degree of cultural transition. Consequently, acculturation has become a dominant framework used to explain disparities among minority groups. As such, we focus on reviewing the evidence on the relationship between acculturation and social exclusion at structural, group and individual levels. For this chapter, Atkinson's (1998) notion of social exclusion is used, which emphasises social relations and ruptures in the social contract rather than resource poverty, and identifies three key features of social exclusion: first, relativity (measuring exclusion by spatially comparing the circumstances of some individuals or communities relative to others at a given time), second, agency (examining the role of some agents and institutions to explain exclusion); and third, dynamics (looking at long-term effects or characteristics of exclusion). Given the complexity of the web to be untangled, we begin by defining the concept of acculturation and examining its historical background. We then move on to examine social exclusion through acculturation lenses focusing on the impact of acculturation on the access to and utilisation of social and health services, and acculturation-related differentials in health outcomes. We finish by examining the implications for public health.

Early research on acculturation emphasised that the acculturation process happens at a group level, with the whole group experiencing structural, cultural, biological, psychological, economic and political changes (for more details see Flannery and colleagues 2001). In addition, it was implied that mutual changes occur in both groups: the dominant group (host society) and the acculturating groups (migrants or refugees). However, due to influences from the host society, most changes occur in the acculturating group (Graves 1967). Nowadays, anthropologists have demonstrated that acculturation occurs at the individual level (Berry 1990a). At this level, acculturation has been termed psychological acculturation, that is, changes in both overt behaviours and covert traits of an individual from a cultural group going through the collective acculturation process (Graves 1967).

However, regardless of the structural level at which the acculturation process occurs, two theoretical models have dominated the literature on acculturation: the unidirectional model (UDM) and the bi-dimensional model (BDM). The UDM assumes that it is not possible to be a fully integrated member of two cultures with two differing sets of cultural values. According to Flannery and colleagues, 'the UDM describes acculturation as the shedding off of an old culture and the taking on of a new culture ... [and] describes only one outcome of acculturation – assimilation' (Flannery *et al.* 2001: 1035). In this respect, the UDM considers acculturation as a linear process where an individual moves from being traditional to assimilating. The problem with this assumption is that the model fails to identify those who are bicultural. Unfortunately, the UDM has predominated research on acculturation and has become the standard view of acculturation (Park and Miller 1921).

In contrast, the BDM measures two cultural orientations – the home and host cultures (Figure 2.3), and assumes that the identifications with traditional and host cultures are independent. This model identifies migrants on four cultural orientations: (1) Traditional, also known as separation (keeps loyalty to traditional culture and does not recognise the host/dominant culture) (Berry and Kim 1988; MacLachlan 1997), (2) Assimilation, also known as 'cultural shift' (Berry 1990b) or the 'melting pot' theory of acculturation (MacLachlan 1997) (rejects traditional culture and fully embraces the host/

dominant culture), (3) Integration, also known as bicultural orientation or cultural incorporation (retains cultural identity at the same time moving to join the dominant society) (MacLachlan 1997) and (4) Marginalisation (rejects traditional culture and fails to connect with the host/dominant culture by exclusion or withdrawal (MacLachlan 1997).

Questions for constructing the instrument (Berry 1998)

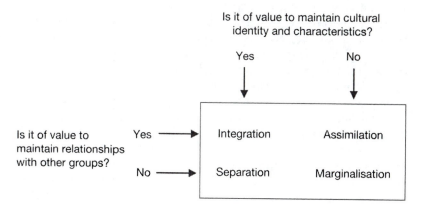

Conceptualising the results

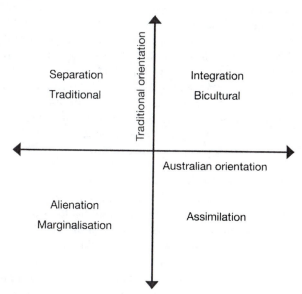

Figure 2.3 Bi-directional model of acculturation

Examining social exclusion through acculturation lenses

Although operationalising and measuring acculturation has become difficult (for example, see detailed discussion of the limitations associated with the application of acculturation theories in Hunt *et al.* 2004; Rudmin 2006), there are many changes to the social context and structure, networks and social support, and communication and language use that occur when two cultural groups come into contact. The process of acculturation can lead to alienation for certain sectors of migrant communities and this may affect their living standards and access to various opportunities. Because migrants bring with them values and norms that substantially deviate from the norms and values of their host populations, they become subject to subtle forms of social exclusion. The principle of the acculturation theory implies that assimilation and integration may allow migrants to understand the strengths and weaknesses of their new environment while separation and marginalisation are more likely to perpetuate the perceptions of discrimination, alienation or disenfranchisement (Leong and Chou 1994). In this sense, acculturation-related changes may increase the effects of poverty, financial stress and social exclusion in different ways. On the one hand, the process of acculturation pushes certain groups of the migrant communities to the margins of the society (i.e. marginalisation), the consequences of which include limited access to, and utilisation of, services, leading to poor social and health outcomes, and lack of necessary life skills required for full participation in employment opportunities and wider social and community networks (López *et al.* 2002).

On the other hand, service providers at the systemic level often fail to recognise that they need to acculturate, and their capacity to provide effective health and social services within and throughout the expanded cultural space becomes limited, leading to one or more of three possible scenarios in service delivery: first, cultural destructiveness – a form of forced assimilation whereby there is only one cultural trend that is acknowledged while purposefully outlawing any other cultural approaches; second, cultural incapacity – where service providers put boundaries on cultural requirements in an equal manner, acknowledging their existence but without engaging them and third, cultural blindness – adopting the 'one approach fits all' theory, whereby the assumption is that people are all alike and what works for one cultural group should also work for the other (see Cross and colleagues 1989 or Renzaho 2002, 2008 for more information). Obtaining data on patterns of service utilisation, service providers' community consultation and engagement with ethnic minorities, quality of services and health outcomes for different cultural groups to identify which ones are most affected, and the extent of service providers' cultural competence would provide information on the level to which a health system is acculturated and the capacity of the health system to meet the needs of all its constituencies. At the individual and group level, migration status and type, population size of the acculturating group, familiarity with host culture, age at migration, personality, and cultural flexibility and characteristics (e.g. how the acculturating group is willing to alter beliefs and traditions to accommodate demands and needs stemming from coming into contact with a new and different culture) combine to determine migrants' level of social exclusion. In their new environment, factors influencing social inclusion through cultural integration and adaptation include the degree of racial tolerance and cultural diversity, support systems, and policies and attitudes toward multiculturalism (Coles 2005).

Some indicators of social exclusion and acculturation: the evidence

Access to and utilisation of primary health care

In Australian primary health care, migrants from a non-English speaking background (NESB) have been found to consistently have longer consultation times, are seven times more likely to attend a medical appointment as a family, and more than twice as likely to attend as a couple, compared with clients of English speaking backgrounds (Renzaho 2007). Increased consultation time, group attendance to an appointment, and increased interpreting cost associated with servicing NESB patients means that this cluster of the population will not receive an adequate level of health care, as these factors are not taken into account in the horizontal fiscal equalisation.[1] Consequently, service providers are not financially equipped to meet these challenges.

However, findings in this area paint an unclear picture. Some studies have reported a negative association between acculturation access to and utilisation of primary health care effect (e.g. Prislin *et al.* 1998) while others found no association (e.g. Shah *et al.* 2006; Marks *et al.* 1987). For example, in their study examining the relationship between the acculturation of Mexican American mothers in Texas and immunisation status of their children between 3 and 24 months of age, Prislin and colleagues (Prislin *et al.* 1998) found that assimilation (moving away from traditional-orientation) contributed to less positive attitudes toward immunisation, a diminished sense of parental responsibility for getting children immunised, and a stronger perception that cost and time were barriers to children's immunisation. After adjusting for potential confounding factors, the authors found that in actual fact assimilation contributed to inadequate children immunisation status, but when the parental attitude toward responsibility and perceived barriers for children's immunisation were added to the model as mediators, the relationship between acculturation and children's immunisation status became insignificant.

In contrast, Shah and colleagues (Shah *et al.* 2006) examined whether maintenance of traditional cultural values was a risk factor for the under-utilisation of colorectal cancer screening among Hispanic populations in the US. Their unadjusted univariate analysis found an inverse relationship between level of acculturation among Hispanics and the likelihood of not having an at-home faecal occult blood test and not having endoscopy in the past year, and the trend was consistent when the analysis was extended for 'the past 5 years'. These results remained consistent when controlling for socioeconomic status (e.g. age, income level, educational level, and poverty threshold) but became non significant when medical history and medical care variables were added to the model. From these findings it is clear that the low use of colorectal screening observed among Hispanics is more due to inadequate access to medical care as a whole rather than their level of acculturation.

Shah and colleagues' findings are similar to those reported by Marks and colleagues (Marks *et al.* 1987). They examined whether cultural factors predict the use of screening examinations (e.g. physical examination from a medical doctor, screening for breast cancer, Pap smear) and found that no dimension of acculturation was strongly or consistently associated with the use of screening examinations, except for language. Although use of the English language was found to be most closely associated with increased screening, most of the effects for language were marginal. The study findings strongly suggest that cultural factors may have little influence on health seeking behaviours and use of preventive health care. These findings were further replicated in a separate study by Solis and colleagues (Solis *et al.* 1990). The latter found that language, but not ethnic identification, was the important predictor of health service utilisation, and that spoken language was the stronger predictor than written language. Nevertheless, the authors caution that the effect of language on screening practices should be considered as an access factor (e.g. improved English ability translates into increased access to services) and not a cultural factor.

Acculturation as a predictor of social issues

Caetano *et al.* (2007) examined the association between acculturation, acculturation stress, drinking and intimate partner violence among Hispanic couples in the US. The authors interviewed 1,392 couples, and distinguished acculturation from acculturation stress. Acculturation measures were concerned with ethnicity of people with whom respondents interacted at church, at parties, and in the neighbourhood; daily use of and ability to speak, read and write English and Spanish; preference for media (books, radio and TV) in English or Spanish; and a series of questions about values thought to be characteristic of the Hispanic lifestyle. In contrast, the measures of acculturation stress assessed issues related to conflicts with family members and friends because of changes in values, problems with communication in English, and adjustment problems associated with participants' ethnic culture. Traditionally-oriented Hispanic males reported more stress than those who adopted US cultural norms and values, and there was a positive association between higher levels of stress (but not acculturation level) and intimate partner violence, but none for drinking. For women, there was an inverse association between acculturation level and acculturation stress, as there was for men, but a positive association between acculturation level (but not acculturation stress) and intimate partner violence, and none for drinking. Although the adoption and adherence to US norms and values translated into less stress, it is possible that the stress accumulated through the process of adaptation to the new country is more likely to explain the increased likelihood of involvement in a violent relationship than drinking.

Hunter *et al.* (2006) examined the relationship between acculturation and driving under the influence among Hispanic population in California. The authors carried out interviews with Hispanic recidivist offenders driving under the influence immediately prior to sentencing, and two years later. The authors found that the less-acculturated members were more likely to report a repeat driving under the influence conviction at two-year follow-up than their highly acculturated counterparts, even after controlling for demographic factors and drinking severity. However, there was no relationship between acculturation level and driving under the influence arrest rates. The study findings suggest that acculturation level is a risk factor for repeat convictions, and programs geared toward reducing multiple driving under the influence convictions need to specifically target the less acculturated in order to increase program effectiveness.

Acculturation-related differentials in health outcomes

Acculturation is associated with changes in chronic disease risk profile. Risk factors and health conditions related to coronary heart disease, cancer, obesity and diabetes differ by acculturation. For example, Kamineni *et al.* (1999) reported that the incidence of gastric carcinoma among Japanese-Americans was three to six times higher that that of American-born whites, and the highest incidence was among Japanese-Americans born in Japan. Despite the higher incidence of gastric cancer reported among Japanese-Americans, it has been estimated that Japanese migrants residing in Hawaii have lower incidence rates of gastric cancer (Hawaiians experience a 50 per cent decrease in stomach cancer risk post migration) but experience increased risk for breast cancer than Japanese in the country of origin (Tsugane 2005).

Similarly, Reed *et al.* (1982) studied a cohort of 4,653 men of Japanese ancestry living in Hawaii. Three acculturation dimensions were used: first, culture of upbringing (e.g. degree of exposure to Japanese influences during childhood, years lived in Japan, age at migration, etc.); second, current cultural assimilation (e.g. degree to which an individual had maintained Japanese culture forms, and included information on ability and frequency of reading and writing Japanese) and third, current social assimilation (e.g. degree to which an individual had maintained contact with Japanese ethnic groups in the community, including information about ethnicity of physicians, friends, employers and co-workers). The study found that there was an inverse relationship between total acculturation scores (1 = most Western; 4 = most traditional) and the prevalence of total coronary heart disease, myocardial infarction and angina. Social assimilation score was also inversely associated with the prevalence of total coronary heart disease, but not myocardial infarction, and angina.

In a critical review of the literature, Perez-Escamilla and Putnik (2007) examined the influence of acculturation on type 2 diabetes and corresponding risk factors, particularly dietary intake, physical activity patterns, smoking and alcohol consumption, and obesity among migrants. Their findings suggest that, among Latinos embracing Western ways, there are both negative and positive outcomes. Negative outcomes include increased obesity risk, suboptimal dietary choices including lack of breast-feeding, low intake of fruits and vegetables, and increased consumption of fats and artificial drinks, smoking and alcohol consumption. Positive outcomes include increased physical activity and a lower likelihood of type 2 diabetes. Other studies have suggested that traditionally-oriented migrants are more likely to have diabetes than their assimilated counterparts (Mainous *et al.* 2006 and Jaber *et al.* 2003). In fact, once diabetes is diagnosed, traditionally-oriented diabetic individuals are more likely to have diabetes complications such as peripheral neuropathy compared with their assimilated counterparts (Mainous *et al.* 2006).

Bhui and colleagues (2005) investigated cultural identity as a risk factor for mental health problems among adolescents in east London's multiethnic community. This was a cross sectional school based survey of a representative sample of 2,790 adolescents from year 7 (11–12 years) and year 9 (13–14 years) attending schools in east London. All the 42 eligible schools were invited to take part in the study and 28 schools agreed to participate. Of the 2,790 adolescents on which data were obtained, 525 (or 20 per cent) were born outside the UK. The sample was composed of white, Pakistani, Indian, Bangladeshi, Mixed race, Black African, Black Caribbean and Black British. The main finding from this study was that integration was healthy and protective against mental health problems. Importantly, integrated cultural identity based on friendship choices was related to fewer mental health problems among adolescents of all ethnic groups. Similarly integration on the basis of friendship choices remained significantly associated with a lower risk of mental health problems after adjusting for socioeconomic indicators, social support from friends, duration of stay in the UK, religion, age, gender and ethnic group. The authors concluded that cultural identity is a more specific risk factor of importance than ethnicity. Similar findings were reported among Ghanaians in the Netherlands. Knipscheer and Kleber (2007) reported that preservation of traditions and maintenance of cultural affiliation were related to lower level mental health problems. They suggest that there are some domains of cultural adaptation that promote mental health of migrants and others that hinder it. They recommend that mental health professionals working with migrants should assess mental health problems as well as establishing the influence of acculturation stress, cultural affiliations and social and economic disadvantage on mental health.

Marino *et al.* (2001) examined the relationship between acculturation and oral health status, oral health knowledge and frequency of dental visits in 147 subjects of Vietnamese background, 18 years or older, living in Melbourne, Australia. Oral health was measured using dental status (decayed, missing and filled surface-DMFS index), recentness of dental visits and preventive dental health knowledge. This study found that assimilation (highly acculturated) had a protective effect against deleterious oral health. Acculturation was associated with all three oral health outcomes measured; dental caries history, knowledge of preventive measures for dental caries and frequency of visits to the dentist. Participants who were assimilated had a lower number of teeth affected with caries history, were more likely to have used oral health services in the twelve months prior to the study, and had a better knowledge of ways of preventing dental caries than traditionally-oriented participants. The study also found that overall, Vietnamese migrants had better dental health than the broader Australian population, suggesting that the oral health outcomes of those who are assimilated are, in fact, relatively even better.

Implications for public health

Research on the relationship between acculturation and its long-term effect of social exclusion has produced mixed findings: some studies have linked acculturation to some deleterious health and social outcomes (Prislin *et al.* 1998; Perez-Escamilla and Putnik 2007); others have reported that acculturation may lead to improved health behaviours and social outcomes (Jaber *et al.* 2003; Perez-Escamilla and Putnik 2007); while few have found no relationship (Marks *et al.* 1987). What is clear is that it has been difficult to compare acculturation studies due to the use of different measures. The acculturation measurement has been dominated by surrogate or proxy measures of acculturation such as length of stay and/or generation (a measure that does not take into account pre-immigration history), language and family values. Some studies did not psychometrically derive their acculturation scales, and in most cases, acculturation was considered as a linear process, where individuals move from one end of the axis (traditional) to the other (assimilation) at a different pace. Few of the studies described above considered acculturation as a bi-dimensional process that conceptually allows for the four types of cultural orientation we described in the introduction (assimilation, marginalisation, traditional and integration). This is particularly important as our recent study on acculturation and obesity found that each of these acculturation types have different health risks. However, the dominant finding across these studies, regardless of the acculturation scale used, is that the benefit of preserving traditional values seems to provide superior health outcomes, suggesting that assimilation is detrimental to health. From a public health perspective, it is clear from these studies that there is a need to identify and preserve traditional practices and culture-based positive attitudes that have health benefits, and incorporate them into health promotion programs.

Notes

1 Horizontal fiscal equalisation is a formula used by the Australian Commonwealth to ensure that States and Territories do not experience disadvantage in their financial capacity to offer equal levels of public goods and services commensurate with their contributed tax effort.

2.10 Discourse, power and exclusion: The experiences of childless women

Gemma E. Carey, Melissa Graham, Julia Shelley and Ann Taket

Throughout culture, motherhood is celebrated while childlessness is promoted as a sorry state. Women without children are ignored unless they are desperately seeking motherhood or are regretfully watching others become mothers and grandmothers. Who is talking about women having viable lives without children of their own? Not many.

(Morell 1994: 1)

While determining the rates of, and reasons for, childlessness is difficult, we know that a general upward trend exists in the number of women who do not mother children in Western countries (Campbell 1985; Seccombe 1991; Ireland 1993; Morell 1994; Bartlett 1996; McAllister and Clark 1998; Gillespie 2001, 2003). Currently, approximately 20 per cent of women fall into this category, whilst historically 10 per cent have represented the norm (Park 2002). This increase relates to an increase in infertility (as a result of delayed parenting, and other factors), but also to an increase in the number of women choosing not to have children, or the voluntarily childless (Seccombe 1991). Current research into the area of voluntary childlessness suggests that significant social exclusion and social connectedness issues may exist for such women.

To date, the conceptual tool of social exclusion has not been applied to the experiences of childless women. By analysing childlessness from a social exclusion perspective, in this chapter we begin to address an important knowledge gap by advancing two areas of thought. First, we provide a new perspective on an emerging social trend; and second, we advance social exclusion theorising by demonstrating that it can be divorced from the economic dimensions of disadvantage with which it is most commonly used. We begin by discussing current literature on childless women which depicts considerable stigma and discrimination issues. Using multiple theoretical perspectives we then attempt to better conceptualise the underlying processes which lead to these negative social experiences. To achieve this we draw on the concepts of discourse, power and social exclusion.

Voluntarily childless women: an emerging social trend

It has been anticipated that 23 per cent of women over the age of 45 in the UK will be childless by 2010 (Gillespie 2003). Although no comparable data exists, such estimates might also apply in countries like Australia. The increasing trend towards childlessness has been interpreted as an effect of rising feminism, increased access to reproductive technology, and women's increased participation in the workforce (Seccombe 1991; Gillespie 2003). Multiple studies (see Houseknecht 1979; Russo 1979; Callan 1986; Heaton *et al.* 1999; Gillespie 2001; Park 2002, 2005) have claimed to have established several common characteristics between the voluntarily childless which support these explanations. These studies have found that women without children are usually tertiary educated, more likely to be employed in professional and managerial positions, and have a high income. With regard to childless couples, both spouses are more likely to have high incomes and a greater flexibility between gender roles (Gillespie 2001; Keizer *et al.* 2007).

The social group(s) in which voluntary childlessness is growing are those which we would expect to see enjoying the benefits of wider social roles afforded by feminism, better reproductive technology, and a less gender-biased workplace. They are not the groups with which we associate disadvantage, as they are well positioned socially and politically, and enjoy full economic participation (both in terms of production and consumption). However, research which has investigated the experiential aspects of childlessness suggests that despite this, women who do not mother are socially disadvantaged. Studies into perceptions and experiences of childless women have found that women who do not have children are a heavily stigmatised and negatively stereotyped group (Letherby 1994, 2000; Letherby and Williams 1999; Gillespie 2000; Park 2002).

Stigma surrounding childlessness has been found to lead to feelings of incompleteness or beliefs that others perceived them as desperate, pitiful and selfish (Letherby 1999). With regard to negative stereotyping, the voluntarily childless tend to be considered socially undesirable, selfish, individualistic, irresponsible, materialistic, under-developed and less caring (Veevers 1974; Gillespie 2000; Park 2002). Park (2002) also found that people expressed a desire for more social distance from voluntary childless people. When compared with parents, Park (2002) argues the voluntary childless are considered less socially desirable, less well adjusted, less nurturant and more autonomous. She contends that voluntary childless women incur a greater degree of stigma than the involuntary, as involuntary childless women embrace the parenting role in theory, if not in practice (Park 2002). While involuntarily childless women are met with pity, voluntarily childless women are likely to be considered selfish (Letherby 1999). These findings are further substantiated by Callan (1986) who found that voluntarily childless individuals were considered more likely to be materialistic, selfish, individualistic and career orientated and that the lives of childfree women were considered less rewarding.

While no research has been conducted explicitly into the area of childlessness and social exclusion, both the findings discussed above and narratives of childless women portray significant connectedness issues. For example, a not uncommon experience for childless women is 'Being with a group of women talking about the apparently inexhaustible topics of their labours, children's eating habits, or teenage rebellion is similar to being in a group of men talking about football. I feel excluded' (Letherby and Williams 1999: 725). This is particularly evident in lay literature (Hutchison (2007: 1): an Australian journalist writes 'I'd like to tell [politicians] about the view of community I have. The one that excludes you if you can't contribute to conversations about nappies and birth choices'.

Social discourses and choosing not to mother

To appreciate how childless women may be socially excluded we must first confront certain characteristics of our current social and political climate (and the discourses which flow from such a climate) in the context of childbearing. Currently, Australian society is characterised by a strong pronatalist ideology which apotheosises motherhood. This glorification of motherhood has consequences for the social dimensions of childbearing, and in turn for choosing not to bear children. Indeed, Park (2002) and Letherby (1999) argue that the stigma and negative evaluations of childless individuals (particularly the voluntarily childless) pertain to, and are derived from, a social environment that continues to be strongly pronatalist. Motherhood and non-motherhood are both private and public performances; dominant discourses, such as pronatalism, therefore profoundly affect how women experience having children, or being voluntarily childless, in both a public and private sense. They affect social interaction and social experience, but also individual attitudes, experiences and emotional responses.

Pronatalist ideology suggests that the 'encouragement of all births [is] conducive to individual, family, and social well-being' (De Sandre 1978: 145 in Park 2005: 357). Pronatalism therefore operates on several levels:

> culturally, when childbearing and motherhood are perceived as 'natural' and central to a woman's identity; ideologically when the motherhood mandate becomes a patriotic, ethnic or eugenic obligation; psychologically when childbearing is identified with the micro level of personal aspirations, emotions and rational decision making ... and on the level of population policy, when the state intervenes, directly or indirectly, in an attempt to regulate the dynamics of fertility.
>
> (Heitlinger 1991: 344–45 in Park 2002: 22)

The political and social climate of pronatalism prevents voluntary childlessness from emerging as an alternative cultural discourse and practice. Furthermore, Park (2002) argues that the political and social emphasis on 'family' values removes the voluntarily childless option from cultural discourse. This is particularly so at present in Australia due to the political emphasis which is currently being placed on population decline, economic viability and national responsibility.

Pronatalism also refracts through other female centred discourses. Our perceptions of motherhood, femininity and feminine identity are all shaped by dominant pronatalist discourses. Gillespie (2000) argues that part of the hegemonic pronatalist doctrine is a dominant 'motherhood discourse'. She contends that in Western culture, motherhood has come to be understood (and presented) as a fixed, natural, fulfilling practice which is central to feminine identity and that 'Constructions of femininity and women's social role have historically and traditionally been contextualised around the practices and symbolism surrounding motherhood' (Gillespie 2000: 223). Powerful discourses, produced through social, political, medical and religious institutions, proliferate the belief that only through motherhood can women be truly fulfilled; mothering and nurturing is what women do, and mothers are what women are (Gillespie 2001). Indeed Russo (1979) suggests that motherhood exists on a different plane from other sex or gender roles for women; it is a mandate that pervades social institutions and individual psyches, and as Gillespie (2001) has noted, the social and cultural discourses of femininity and motherhood are particularly slow to change.

Similarly, Hird and Abshoff (2003: 347) state that the 'symbolic configuration of women as mothers extends beyond the familial boundary to support an ideology of gender that specifies women's "nature" as sexually reproductive'. Nevertheless, Letherby (1994) draws attention to what is possibly a contradiction, or perhaps irony, of the dominant motherhood discourse. Despite the sanctity of motherhood and the judgements made about those who choose not to mother, many would argue that motherhood itself has had little status in Western society.

Due to these prevailing social discourses women who choose not to have children challenge dominant perceptions of female identity and femininity. Concurrent with this, they have become constructed as a morally deviant 'other' in contemporary Australian society. Park (2002: 22) suggests that this moral objectification is twofold: 'the deviance of the voluntarily childless lies not only in the fact that they do not have children, but primarily, and especially for women, in the fact that they do not want them'. Similarly, Letherby (1999: 230) found that people perceived a lack of desire to mother as deviant and abnormal because it 'transgressed cultural images of femininity, of nurturing and self-sacrifice, associated with motherhood'.

These pronatalist discourses represent a dominant feature of Australian society. They are normative in that they dictate standards of behaviour and shape social norms. But how have pronatalist discourses gained such social legitimacy?

Discourse and power

We cannot speak of discourse, and certainly not of dominant or normative discourses, without raising the subject of power. Power is what makes discourses hold true and renders them dominant and normative. Foucault's (1980) concept of power is particularly useful for understanding the relationships between discourse, power and exclusion. In understanding how discourses and power operate, we may begin to appreciate the relations which are the underlying root of disadvantage.

Under a Foucauldian conceptualisation of power, power is ubiquitous. It flows throughout daily life, rather than being held in a central locale (as the Marxist tradition would suggest) that 'Power must be analyzed as something which circulates ... And not only do individuals circulate between its threads: they are always in a position of simultaneously undergoing and exercising this power' (Foucault 1980: 98). Foucault's conception of power is also productive in nature; it formulates discourse and knowledge which is given legitimacy through institutions (Dreyfus and Rabinow 1982). Thus, just as state power is ubiquitous, so too are the discourses which flow from it.

Population policies, which promote procreation-based answers to economic and social problems, imbue pronatalist discourses with the authority of the state and other social institutions. Such discourses therefore gain substantial legitimacy and are able to regulate childbearing behaviour and attitudes at both a population and individual level by establishing social norms. Such discourses also have strong moral undertones which serve to further regulate the behaviour of individuals and populations. It is worth noting that discursive power is therefore both an individual and a totalising power – it dictates appropriate behaviour on a population level, but also singles out individuals that transgress social norms (Foucault 1980).

State power, in conjunction with medical and religious institutions, legitimises pronatalist discourse. Through this process such discourses become normative in so much as they establish social norms and expected behaviours. However, in dictating certain practices as normal, others by virtue become considered 'abnormal', or deviant. It is in this sense that we can begin to appreciate the underlying processes that lead to the social exclusion of childless women.

Social exclusion

Social exclusion has emerged as a term to conceptualise disadvantage and the processes which cause disadvantage. It derives from a lack of choice and sociability and is often linked with notions of stigma, vulnerability and marginalisation, as these phenomena are often associated with the breakdown of social cohesion. In conjoining discussions of power and discourse with social exclusion we are able to better appreciate the processes which underpin stigma, discrimination and social connectedness issues of childless women.

De Haan (1998) argues that social exclusion has two defining characteristics; first, it focuses attention on the fact that deprivation is multidimensional (and can include aspects of material poverty and/or social deprivation); and second, that it enables a focus on the relations and processes which cause deprivation. Subsequently, it is useful in analysing 'societal links, social participation, and interrelated issues such as the disadvantages of impoverished social networks, which can disrupt social bonds and lead to social isolation or lack of social integration' (Arthurson and Jacobs 2004: 30). Whilst social exclusion is often used as an alternative term for poverty, material poverty is not a requirement for social exclusion.

The theory of social exclusion therefore allows insight into the social relations, processes and institutions which both enable society to function, but are the underlying root of deprivation (de Haan 1998). It is in this way that social exclusion is often used to conceptualise and/or analyse the social structures (such as race, gender and class) or policy environments which affect disadvantaged populations (see for example, Colley and Hodkinson 2001; Martin 2004; Horsell 2006). This focus upon social relations and institutions, however, is also useful for understanding how individuals may be disadvantaged due to their incongruence with social norms. In the previous section we outlined how pronatalist discourses are made legitimate by state power, and come to pervade daily life, normalising certain practices and making others 'deviant'. In becoming society's 'deviant' others, childless women become stigmatised, discriminated against and ultimately socially excluded. Indeed, Weedon (1987 in Letherby 1999) contends that maintaining a dominant ideology, such as pronatalism, requires the marginalising of experiences which seek to redefine it. Weedon's comment contextualises the experiences of stigma described by childless women, and further illustrates how childless women are socially excluded due to normative pronatalist discourses.

Reidpath *et al.* (2005) link stigma with social value and the existence of social exclusion. They suggest that social exclusion relates to the ability of individuals' to be involved in reciprocal exchange. If an individual is considered deficient in a particular area, or is stigmatised, they are perceived to have no means by which they may 'give back'. Subsequently, individuals become excluded from social relations because social tensions are eased when such individuals are not included. In the case of childless women, these women may be considered to have little social value due to dominant pronatalist ideologies.

Current research suggests that exclusion of childless women is more complex than simply being denied social participation. Our pronatalist environment leads some women to subvert their 'deviant' identities, or alternatively to exclude themselves as 'the context of continuing pronatalism ... requires many childless individuals to engage in information control and stigma management techniques, tailored to particular audiences, to manage their deviant identities' (Park 2005: 372). Many women also feel the need to divert attention away from their voluntarily childfree identities (Letherby and Williams 1999; Letherby 2002; Park 2002). For example, Letherby (1999; 2002) found that childfree women felt it was easier to say that they hadn't made a decision, and keep their 'status' and experiences hidden, while Morell (1994: 305) notes that women must 'constantly engage in acts of subversion if they pursue goals that are not stereotypically "feminine"'.

Based on the limited research available, the above analysis suggests that there is likely to be a considerable (and complex) social exclusion issue for women without children. This chapter represents a first attempt to explore this issue in a scholarly forum, but much more extensive work on this issue is still needed. The growing magnitude, yet minority and marginalised status of this group of women suggest that this is a deficit that needs to be addressed.

2.11 Over 60 and beyond ... the alienation of a new generation: exploring the alienation of older people from society

Annemarie Nevill

The global phenomenon of population ageing brings with it a myriad of challenges for many older people, including major economic, health and social impacts. Modernisation and globalisation have created major and often pervasive sociocultural changes, which are now evident in most developed and developing countries. As a result, traditional values are breaking down, such as family cohesion and traditional care and support, and in its wake, those over 60 now inadvertently form a *new generation* of marginalised people; hence the alienation of this newly-formed generation of those aged 60 and above.

Since the twentieth century, the population across the globe is ageing at an unparalleled rate. This is how the 'ageing population' is commonly defined, and coupled with an incremental growth in longevity, the burden of chronic diseases correspondingly increase. Given the consequences that population ageing bring to each stratum of society, there are often reactive rather than proactive responses to human ageing from macro, meso and micro levels of society. This is largely a consequence of ageist reactions to ageing itself.

Due to factors surrounding the complexities of the ageing population, in recent years it had been recognised that there is a case for an international convention on the rights of older people (Tang and Lee 2006). As they age, people become devalued and lose their rights as active members of society. In a world where neglect and violation of older people's rights are common, to what extent do these factors contribute to the feelings of alienation of this age group?

This chapter will examine factors which have historically led to this *new generation* being marginalised from society. Given the exponential growth of the ageing population in Western countries, it is envisaged that the social exclusion or alienation of older people is an issue of great public health significance, in particular, contributing to an escalation of the burden of mental health, depression and general well-being of this group. What was the 'golden age' for many is now emerging as the era of the 'black dog'.

Factors such as a breakdown of tradition, materialism, gender issues, ageing as a social justice issue, and the acceleration of the vulnerability, fear and dependency of older people will be discussed in the light of their contribution to the alienation of this new generation of older people.

A nostalgic lament for younger days

> I wish I could go back to the beautiful days of my life ... remember other
> sweet moments and faces which would erase, albeit for a moment, the
> images which come back to my sense [...] Why can't I fly away on the
> wonderful wings of memory?
>
> (Schwarz-Bart *et al.* 1966, cited in de Souza 2002: 155)

This is a passage, a lament for younger days by an older Caribbean woman,
Mariotte, confined to a nursing home, a character deprived of her identity, with
nostalgic words reflecting the plight so often felt by older people. Philosopher
Isaiah Berlin (1965 cited in Jalving n.d.) romanticised nostalgia and alienation,
with the following:

> It is nostalgia, it is reverie, it is intoxicating dreams, it is sweet melan-
> choly and bitter melancholy, solitude, the sufferings of exile, the sense of
> alienation, roaming in remote places, especially in the East, and in
> remote times, especially the Middle Ages.
>
> (Jalving n.d.)

For older people, the term 'alienation' holds no such haunting reverie, but is
useful in explaining the waves of discontent that permeate a society dominated
by the determinants of modernisation: technology, commercialism, materialism, competitiveness and individualism. These may be conducive to maintaining a somewhat meaningful link between most people, but for older people,
these can often contribute to distancing them from others who are, for
example, technologically savvy. Whereby technology, such as using a computer
at home, plays an important role in the lifestyle of those aged between 45–64
years, older cohorts tend to not have had the same experiences with information technology as their younger counterparts have had (Australian Institute
of Health and Welfare [AIHW] 2007) and subsequently are excluded from this
rapidly expanding and prominent characteristic of modernisation. However, as
older people learn about computers via suitably designed training programs for
this cohort, this will ultimately improve life satisfaction, independence and the
development of social networks of this group (Broady *et al.* 2008).

How has alienation been historically recognised in the literature, and what
meanings have been ascribed to it? Hegel (cited in Schacht 1971) first elevated
the term 'alienation' to a position of philosophical importance, and it has
since been widely utilised in a range of inquiry dealing with social life, values
and human well-being. According to Keniston (1972), existentialists have
suggested that human existence over the last century has become dis-
connected because there is an inherent lack of purpose to life, which results in
meaning being artificially manufactured by humans in the process of existence,
often via material means. However, most theorists concur that the fundamental characteristics of alienation involve feelings of loss, powerlessness,

meaninglessness and estrangement from self and society (Seeman 1959). This reflects Marx's conception of alienation, which ranges from the individual being indifferent to being 'alienated' or to attributing certain feelings towards feeling lonely and powerless (Archibald 1978). These latter meanings are often echoed in older people's lives.

Controversies in the literature have evolved over the significance and purpose of the state of alienation in one's life; is alienation (or in this case, solitude) a positive contributor to a person's life journey, or a state that is deleterious to one's health? In an example of this debate, Gotesky (1965: 226) maintained that 'alienation is a negatively inescapable state that can be transcended only in solitude or else we cope "in the walled prison of loneliness"'. Added to this, few people have been able to live in a state of solitude, and 'our pure self has been diluted by others, and that we are social creatures with an innate capability and desire to connect to others with which we share this earth' (Gotesky 1965: 237). Barakat (1969: 2) added to these views when he explored the behavioural consequences of alienation, viewing 'man (as) not only powerless in the face of external conditions; he is also powerless in the face of himself'.

In 1966, Colette wrote that there are days when 'solitude is a heavy wine that intoxicates you', on other days 'when it is a poison that makes you beat your head against the wall' (139). This exemplifies the two sides of this debate. Koch (1994), however, discerned the difference between solitude and alienation by identifying five primary virtues linked to solitude: freedom, attunement to self, and attunement to nature, reflective perspective and creativity.

There has been an emergence of those who recognise the centrality of 'mind, body and spirit' as highlighted in the spiritual literature, whereby states of solitude, mindfulness and other meditative practices do not lead to an impenetrable isolation of people, but are means of negotiating the dilemmas of the self within a society, which is at times inclusive, and at other times exclusive. In this event, solitude becomes a search for the sacred.

When solitude is more about a perception of unwarranted social exclusion, this is experienced more so by older people. Dean (1961) defined alienation as having three major components: powerlessness, normlessness and social isolation; not surprisingly, he found a small positive correlation between alienation and advancing age. Durant and Christian (1990) conducted a study of 200 older clients of metropolitan senior service centres to determine the correlation between selected socioeconomic variables (ethnicity, education, income, health, living arrangement, church work and volunteer work) with four subtypes of alienation. Health, ethnicity, education and income were found to be the strongest predictors of alienation, with those participants from lower socioeconomic backgrounds and with lower health ratings experiencing higher levels of alienation.

Hawthorne (2006) further proposed three key theories of social support, and based on these theories, social isolation, emerging from a 'poor fit between an individual and their social milieu' (526) is defined as 'living without companionship, having low levels of social contact, little social support, feeling separate from others, being an outsider, isolated and suffering loneliness' (521). Clearly, as they age, the elderly face a series of life events, such as death of a spouse, family members and friends, declining health and changes in cognition, retirement and associated lifestyle stages.

Havens *et al.* (2004) compared predictors of social isolation and loneliness for very old urban and rural adults, and found that a number of factors emerged, such as the importance of health and social factors to the social isolation and loneliness of these adults; factors predicting social isolation and loneliness were living alone and low life satisfaction; and that different health problems (such as the presence of multiple chronic illnesses), housing and service options have different impacts upon social isolation and loneliness. These factors should be considered in the development of appropriate integrative health and social policies.

Gardner *et al.* (1999) stated the most important predictors of social isolation in the Australian veteran community were poor health and significantly poor self-rated health. From a gender perspective, men are more likely to be isolated than women, and widowed women tend to be more socially active than widowed men. Clearly, this impacts upon how people experience feelings of alienation as they age (Rokach *et al.* 2007).

Breakdown of tradition ... global transitions and care for those who are ageing

It is no surprise global ageing has and will continue to bring with it different sets of challenges. Over the next 50 years, ageing is the most significant population change projected to occur globally, and this trend is unlikely to be reversed (AIHW 2007); related to this is a fragile financial security for older people. Given changes to family forms and family role obligations, the family's responsibility for support of its elderly members has changed over the generations shaped by shifts in culture, modernisation, globalisation, changing social and family arrangements, migration, acculturation and public policies. These, coupled with deficiencies in public retirement policies and support programs, mean older people are less likely to be economically and socially secure hence be able to cope across other areas in their lives. It has also been speculated that although in Western societies 'baby boomers' will bring change to demographics, they will be more likely to live alone, live in outer suburbs and tend to have fewer children than their older counterparts from previous generations (Kutza 2005).

Older people who live alone are at risk of experiencing loneliness and social isolation and are more likely to need outside assistance in the case of illness. Transport can be problematic for older people, particularly given that driving ability and access to a motor vehicle licence later in life can enhance their independence. Transport availability is critical for many older people's ability to access, for example, health services (AIHW 2007). With policy shifts towards independence, 'ageing well' and remaining at home, this is indeed problematic.

We must not forget the dichotomy between many who live alone who cherish their independence and wish to remain in their homes (Yeh and Lo 2004), and those who wish to maintain strong social networks and do not like living alone. Explanations for this include fear of institutionalisation, deterioration and loss of self.

Although not the focus of this chapter, it is interesting to note that younger people now growing up in traditional cultures are experiencing identity confusion, and their future will be very different from what their parents and grandparents experienced (Arnett 2002).

Ageing in an ageist society

It is important to observe that emerging dichotomies explain what it is to be 'old' in the twenty-first century. All in all, it is not surprising that to anticipate ageing raises fear and anxiety, as it marks a time of loss and burden (Baltes and Carstensen 2003), but on the other side of the coin, being older can be a time of 'growth, vitality, contentment and striving' (82). The proponents of successful ageing state it can be a time where most people can live their lives in relatively good health. Ageing here is seen as a 'dialectic between self-actualisation and self-alienation' (84). Yet, the negativity of ageing continues to endure. In most Western cultures older people are marginalised and socially excluded on the basis of age. In this throwaway society, there is the promotion of 'the slow social death of the elderly by isolating and marginating them' (Palermo 2001: 219). So those who are 'ageing' become socially excluded from dominant constructs of value and esteem, as at the crux of this process ageing is a reminder of mortality and death (Biggs 2004; Martens *et al.* 2005).

What are some of the implications of ageing in an ageist society? Older people tend to suffer the consequences of age discrimination, and these profoundly negative perspectives result in an inherent sense of exclusion for many older people (Harding 2005). By virtue of their age and the state of their senescence and 'decrepitude', their lives become fragmented as they are symbolically ejected by today's throwaway society and metaphorically enter the status of non-personhood (Ng 1998). According to Russell (1951: 106):

> Collective fear stimulates herd instinct, and tends to produce ferocity toward those who are not regarded as members of the herd.

The disenfranchisement in old age is a denial of equal dignity, and is deeply entrenched in the social fabric from which social attitudes are woven (Harding 2005). Bytheway (2005) labelled old age as 'a construction that has a certain popular utility in sustaining ageism within societies that need scapegoats' (119). One of the major trends and challenges of this ageing population is that older people are now viewed in terms of the demands they place rather than the contributions they make. This will become more evident with the acceleration of ageing predicted to continue globally (National Institute on Aging and National Institutes of Health 2007; Kilcannon *et al.* 2005). What leads to intergenerational conflict is further fuelled by the continuing decrease in the relative size of the labour force participation and a reduction in fertility rates contrasted with increasing life expectancy (Australian Bureau of Statistics 2008).

Contemporary Western cultures have a narcissistic obsession of youth, although this becomes yet another facet of social masquerading. This is explained by Baudrillard (1993) who outlined that such

> representations become masks that disguise basic reality, and that these representations hide an inner emptiness. So the implication is that older age has become empty, and depends upon representations from earlier parts of the life course. People attempt to slow down their ageing selves in order to win a reprieve from a 'marginal and ultimately asocial slice of life'.
>
> (Baudrillard cited in Biggs 2004: 48).

In sharp contrast to this normative social phenomenon is that often older people no longer value the years they have lived, without which they have 'no history, no genuine self' (Andrews 1999: 316). Simone de Beauvoir put it so succinctly:

> When we look at the image of our own future provided by the old we do not believe it: an absurd inner voice whispers that that will never happen to us – when that happens it will no longer be ourselves that it happens to.
>
> (de Beauvoir 1970: 3)

The old as the 'other'

Canales (2000) proposed a theoretical framework of how we connect with 'others'. Use of exclusionary othering perpetuates an assumed 'membership' offered to the young by dominant cultures. This acts to sustain the power within relationships for domination, oppression and subordination, taking advantage of stigmatising features characteristic of age, gender, ethnicity and class backgrounds (Bond *et al.* 2004). Interestingly though, some individuals may be unaware that they are the excluded 'other', and are therefore oblivious to their 'exclusion'. With this, it is important to be reminded that the exclusionary/inclusionary divide is in fact a social artefact, whereby we may be included in some groups, but excluded from others. It is often those who are least empowered, such as older people, who have been stigmatised and condemned, particularly by those who believe that older people have surpassed their 'use-by-dates', and are an increasing burden at many levels. They are perceived as different from the status quo who dictate social norms; the visibility of their age renders them invisible. The theory of 'inclusionary othering' is a way to transform and strengthen relationships. Its 'practices attempt to use power to create transformative relationships in which the consequences are consciousness raising, sense of community, shared power, and inclusion' (Canales 2000: 25). Exclusionary practices are restrictive, and based on sameness; inclusionary othering expands the boundaries of its membership, which is based on difference.

Culture, gender and age – the double-edged sword for the already marginalised

Ageism and alienation are sociocultural constructs. Yun and Lachman (2006) detected beliefs about ageing varied by culture, age and gender. Women and men experience loneliness quite differently, and married men are especially vulnerable to interpersonal isolation (Rokach *et al.*. 2007). AIHW (2007) reported that unmarried older men who live alone are at risk of experiencing social isolation, because unmarried women typically report stronger social networks than unmarried men (Yeh and Lo 2004). Meeks *et al.* (1999) identified that women around the globe typically live longer than men, often without the economic resources to maintain independence.

Van Der Geest (1994) presented the paradoxical situation of elderly people still engaged in social activities but still experiencing loneliness, as what they find most valuable in their lives is to have others listen to their advice and wisdom. Loss of respect for them constitutes loneliness. Sung and Kim (2003) proposed recognition of cultural forms of respect and their changing expressions need further exploration.

In traditional societies such as Japan, intergenerational support systems in later life are based on the cultural value of *oya koh koh* (filial obligation), affecting the nature of support from adult children to older parents (Kobayashi 2000). Kim and Kim (2003) showed, however, that elderly as well as younger generations put more value on two-way intergenerational relations based on mutual care and assistance, rather than simply following the traditional norm of filial piety.

The impact of alienation upon the mental health of older people

Hawthorne (2006) has associated social isolation with poorer health status, and refers to living without social connectedness, having an absence of significant others to turn to in times of crisis, reduced life meaning and satisfaction, well-being and community participation. Those who are socially isolated are higher consumers of health care services, have poor outcomes from acute treatment, and tend towards a higher rate of mental illness including dementia and premature death. Hedelin *et al.* (2001) demonstrated that mental health status has major implications for older people's sense of alienation as well as shaping the summation of their lives in general (AIHW 2007).

Han *et al.* (2007) explored the issues of acculturative stress and depression for predominantly first-generation immigrants, and found that these were alleviated by social support, particularly from their family members. Similarly, the work of health advocates to build service provision of culturally appropriate and accessible medical and social services and to strengthen social support networks assisted the reduction of both mental illness and perceptions of loneliness in Somali elders in East London. An elevated sense of belonging to the community was associated with improved mental health of Somali men who migrated to East London and reduced levels of mental illness and feelings of loneliness (Silveira and Allebeck 2001).

So, which comes first – alienation, or mental illness, such as depression? One answer to this is there is a strong juxtaposition between mental illness being one of the leading causes of the total burden of disease and injury in Australia (Australian Bureau of Statistics 2008) and ageing being the most significant population change projected to occur both globally and in Australia. Given this, research into social gerontology and mental health needs directed and sustainable focus on these global health problems.

Alienation and social exclusion as a human rights violation and social justice issue

Older people are vulnerable to human rights violations as they become dependent upon the care of others (Harding 2005). They are at risk of a culture of abuse perpetrated by individuals, organisations and institutions, and via policy systems that are designed to uphold the dignity and safety of older people, but can fail to do so. These actions further alienate the victim. Tang and Lee (2006) argued that the introduction and ratification of an international convention on the rights of older people is long overdue. These authors proposed that international Non-Government Organisations and human rights advocates should work together toward creating such a convention, which needs to be clearly articulated and supported across all public policy debates (Cassel 2001).

A construct of 'successful ageing'

Across the lifespan, society needs to inculcate adaptation and hence resilience from an early age (Consedine *et al.* 2005). Successful ageing, as we understand it, is based upon the concept of adaptation, whereby an individual's progress is measured by the extent to which he or she conforms to the needs of the existing society (Andrews 1999). However, this concept is debatable, as how does this shape the needs of the individual?

According to Palermo (2001: 217), if people are able to maintain 'a sense of personal identity and continuity', then ageing is likely to be successful. However, Torres (2003) discusses the debate that universally acceptable definitions of what constitutes successful ageing is lacking, and our understanding of 'successful ageing' has been based on the Western, middle-class construct of success which is limited across different cultures, traditions and personal values orientations.

Within contemporary capitalist consumer societies the physical appearance of the ageing body has rarely been venerated. As in earlier times, wealth, power and youth remain the main source of reverence; hence, most stereotypes of ageing are negative. There is a blurring of life stages with a shift towards generational sameness, as ageing is valued as successful to the extent that it is 'youthful' (Biggs *et al.* 2006).

Von Faber *et al.* (2001) presented an interesting qualitative model of successful ageing, and factors which contribute to the goal of overall well being. These factors include not only adaptation to life events, but that physical and cognitive functioning are viewed as a way for older people to function on a 'desired social level', with 'social contacts' also contributing to the desired result of successful ageing (2007). It is generally recognised that the 'gold standard' for successful ageing is difficult to both quantify and qualify, and that further research needs to be conducted to explore the intricacies of what it means to age 'well'. Added to this, the work that researchers such as Kessler and Staudinger (2007) have conducted on the potential of intergenerational social interaction needs to be explored further to counter the current trend of intergenerational conflict, particularly when older people are perceived to be a burden at many different levels.

Conclusion

We must continue to question the differential treatment of people based on age, as this not only constitutes a denial of the wisdom and other special qualities of later life but is a fundamental denial of the human rights of older people.

More needs to be understood about ageing including further exploration of personal and cultural values, orientations, expectations and needs across all generations to alleviate the marginalisation and alienation of all groups in society. This is the beginning of a new road towards the celebration and assertion of difference with dignity.

Dedication

For my mother, Maria Mileo Gallichio – all my work done for you. I wish I could go back to the beautiful days of my life with you.

Acknowledgement

I would like to acknowledge Dr Megan Moore's great inspiration and loving encouragement to explore the alienation of older people.

2.12 'Exclusion by inclusion': bisexual young people, marginalisation and mental health in relation to substance abuse

Erik Martin and Maria Pallotta-Chiarolli

Introduction: exclusion by inclusion of 'X files'

> It's like we're the X-files or something. We're not straight A files or gay B files. It's like we mess up their [gay and straight communities'] tidy sex files. But that means they make you feel like you're messed up yourself, as if there's no way their filing system is what's really fucked.
>
> (Marita, adolescent research participant)

This chapter demonstrates the powerful workings of bifurcation in dominant youth health paradigms and discourses that exclude, marginalise or demand assimilation by 'X file' young people, such as Marita above, who are situated on the borders, in-between or beyond the 'straight A files' or 'gay B files'. We will draw from our semi-structured interview research that explored the lived realities and mental health needs of 30 Australian bisexual adolescents and young adults (aged 15 to 25 years), and 15 youth health/community service providers (see also Martin 2007; Pallotta-Chiarolli 2005a, 2006, 2010). In particular, we will focus on substance abuse as exemplifying some of the implications and costs of such exclusions, isolation, conformity and marginalisation.

Probyn's (1996) term, 'outside belonging', can be used to describe the movement between and beyond sexual binaries to a recognition of sexual fluidity, intermixture and heterogeneity. Bisexual-identifying or bisexual-behaving young people are both 'outside' (excluded from) heteronormative and 'homonormative' constructs of sexual binaries, and yet 'belonging' (included) in the sense that they may 'pass' as a 'normal' heterosexual or 'normal' homosexual. Subsequently, they are 'outside' (excluded from) the dominant constructs of gay community and heterosexual society in Australia while simultaneously 'belonging' (included) due to their same-sex and opposite-sex attractions and relationships.

It needs to be stated that our research and discussion in this chapter are not positioned in opposition to or undermining hard-fought gay and lesbian identities, communities and civil rights. Indeed, many gay and lesbian adolescents and young people are still experiencing extreme levels of discrimination, marginalisation and exclusion, particularly in schools, resulting in high levels of mental health issues and risk-taking behaviours (Pallotta-Chiarolli

2005b; Cabaj 2005; McCabe *et al.* 2003; Hughes and Eliason 2002). The effects of 'homonormativity' in relation to bisexuality and sexual fluidity must be explored as a reflection of the wider socio-political heteronormative need to neatly categorise and divide persons into either/or sexualities, genders and relationship models in order to exclude, control and manipulate. The success and power of these heteronormative systems of exclusion, control and manipulation are evident in the internal exclusionary and divisive measures applied to bisexuality and sexual fluidity within gay and lesbian communities in order to construct a united front against such powerful forces (McLean 2008). The power of heteronormativity on bisexual young people is evident in the following account of a young research participant:

> I became quite depressed, quite anxious about my sexuality ... I was crying continuously, I couldn't sleep. This went on for about two weeks. I had to go and stay with my dad because I wasn't eating, I wasn't showering, ... I couldn't look after myself, I couldn't function. And I know that it did stem from me questioning my sexuality, and I thought it was the end of the world ... I kept telling myself 'Michelle, you're supposed to be straight, men and women are supposed to be together, there's not supposed to be anything else.'
>
> (Michelle)

As exemplified by bisexual adolescents and young people in our research, as well as their counsellors and youth workers, recent studies are pointing to higher rates of anxiety, depression and other mental health concerns among Australian bisexual-identifying adolescents and young people as compared to homosexual and heterosexual young people (Jorm *et al.* 2002). There appears to be a strong link between these findings and the under-representation and misrepresentation of bisexuality in Australian schools, queer communities, and health policy, programs, research and services (Pallotta-Chiarolli 2006; McLean 2001). In their review of 'scholarly attention previously given to mental health among bisexual individuals when compared to homosexual and heterosexual individuals', Dodge and Sandfort found that the number of articles that present 'relevant information specific to bisexuals in terms of mental health is a miniscule proportion of the published literature on sexual orientation and mental health' (2007: 41; see also Diamond 2008).

Many educational and health organisations focusing on same-sex attracted young people gain funding for projects that appear to be inclusive of bisexual young people by incorporating bisexuality as a category in their 'gay, lesbian, bisexual, transgender (GLBT)' project outlines and submissions, but they do not follow through with bisexually-specific recommendations, outcomes and services for youth. Heath refers to this as the 'silent B' in much GLBT research: 'as gay and lesbian issues have begun to reach Australian health policy machinery, bisexual people have been almost completely excluded' (Heath 2005: pages unnumbered; see also Russell and Seif 2002).

There are many of these examples of what we call 'exclusion by inclusion' in international health research (Parsons *et al.* 2006; Cabaj 2005; Hughes and Eliason 2002). In 1998, Garofalo *et al.* found lesbian, gay and bisexual (LGB) young people were three and a half times as likely to have attempted suicide during the past year and more likely to engage in other risk behaviours such as alcohol and drug abuse than were heterosexual youth. Although it was noted that 78 per cent of the sample identified as bisexual, there was no comment upon how this high proportion might affect the findings. Ten years later, 'exclusion by inclusion' research based within the sexual bifurcation discourse is still being undertaken and published, albeit more often problematising these research methods and sexual binary systems of classification. For example, Hatzenbuehler *et al.* (2008) explored alcohol use among LGB and heterosexual young adults that demonstrated higher rates of alcohol consumption among what they call 'nonheterosexual' young men and women. They concluded that 'minority stress' would add to the consumption of alcohol among LGB adolescents and young adults 'in order to cope with stress related to having a stigmatized identity' (2008: 88). However, as they conceded, they did not analyse their data to determine how different types and levels of 'minority stress' within the LGB grouping may have impacted upon individual alcohol consumption levels. After acknowledging that the combination of 'individuals with same-sex and both-sex orientations ... obscured important within-group differences among LGB students', the researchers recommend that future studies 'should oversample bisexuals, especially in light of recent findings' that they are at higher risk 'for substance use and abuse' (2008: 88).

The above examples illustrate that the importance of undertaking research with invisibilised or marginalised populations in order to inform health policy, programming and practice has been increasingly espoused, and yet this connection has largely remained ignored in relation to bisexual young people. Research in the US and UK has begun to address 'exclusion by inclusion' concerns in relation to bisexual youth health. Bisexual youth have been found to have higher rates of suicide attempts, substance abuse and overall health risks (Ford and Jasinski 2006; Warner *et al.* 2004; Eisenberg and Wechsler 2003; Goodenow *et al.* 2002; Robin *et al.* 2002; Udry and Chantala 2002).

In Australia, the importance of bi-specific health research and service provision became evident when Jorm *et al.* (2002) publicised their alarming findings into bisexual youth health, as presented earlier in this chapter. In the same year, the Australian Medical Association released a position statement on 'Sexual Diversity and Gender Identity' that includes statement 4.3 acknowledging how recent studies report that bisexual people have worse mental health than their homosexual or heterosexual counterparts (Australian Medical Association 2002). This was accredited to more adverse life events and less positive support from family and friends, as well as possibly being at greater risk of sexually transmitted infections due to a lack of targeted health promotion activities. In 2003, the Victorian Ministerial Advisory Committee on Gay and Lesbian Health noted the lack of research on the sexual health needs of 'bisexually active' people. However, it proposed 'nothing to rectify this situation' (Heath 2005: pages unnumbered). Rather, it called for the establishment of a health and well-being policy and research unit which would 'focus on gay and lesbian health but address bisexual, trans and intersex health issues in so far as they overlap with those of gay men and lesbians' (Ministerial Advisory Committee on Gay and Lesbian Health 2003: 149). Here we see 'exclusion by inclusion' operating at the level of health policy where notions of overlap are deployed as signifying inclusion while in reality meaning continued exclusion.

In the rest of this chapter, we will explore the implications of 'exclusion by inclusion' from the heterosexual mainstream, gay and lesbian communities, and health services on bisexual adolescents' and young people's mental health in relation to substance abuse. This is in line with a 'settings-based approach' to substance use and risk management as 'young people's drug use always takes place within specific cultural settings where the setting itself influences the ways in which risks are experienced' (Duff 2003: 286). It will become evident that exclusion from and/or inclusion within both heterosexual mainstream groups and gay/lesbian groups and their health and community services are significant in understanding and addressing bisexual young people's substance abuse.

The links between social excluson by inclusion of bisexual youth in heterosexual groups and substance use

A sense of isolation in relation to the heteronormative mainstream was commonly referred to by the adolescent and young adult participants in our research. There were several instances where substance abuse was seen as a way of coping with discrimination and marginalisation within families, from heterosexual peers and within heteronormative institutions such as schools. Sam talked about his use of anti-depressants, although this was a licit, maintenance dose, and related it to 'not feeling that there's any comfortable place to rest in terms of my identity'. He also gave details about his use of alcohol and marijuana in relation to bisexual young people's mental well-being:

> Bisexual people have to be on their toes, you know, there's no sense of belonging, ... they're not expected to be anywhere ... With alcohol and marijuana, I think it's more about a sense of numbing because ... there's often a lot of problems that they don't have the tools to address, and ... I think there's a lot of reasons to want to repress that [being bisexual and belonging nowhere].

Victoria stated the following in relation to her 'alcoholism':

I wouldn't fall prey to alcoholism because of my sexuality. It would be more due to loneliness, which is a result of having not as much emotional support from my family ... to kind of escape the reality of being home.

Geographical isolation and living in a rural environment may have an exacerbating effect on the lack of social support and subsequent substance abuse for a bisexual young person, although there is no available literature in this specific area. Michelle, a young bisexual participant who was part of a rural community for a significant proportion of her life, commonly referred to difficulties in growing up and being quite isolated in relation to her sexual orientation, support groups and health services:

I think I'm quite passionate when it comes to people living in rural areas ... I think it's more difficult to get access to even social groups and support groups. ... I never had access to any of that ... it was just nothing.

Michelle explained how there was little to do, and 'pubs' became a main focus in socialising and feeling included within this heteronormative environment:

there was no way at that stage I felt I could talk to my friends that I was socialising with then, so it was much easier to have a drink, and just try and relax that way and forget about it [bisexuality] ... I suppose drinking – maybe a little bit of marijuana ... That was just a way for me to ease through some of the Friday/Saturday/Thursday nights.

Even when bisexual young people were able to socialise with gay and lesbian young people, away from heteronormative spaces and homophobic surveillance, there was often a strong internalised awareness of having been rejected by heteronormative mainstream spaces and institutions which forced them to seek out alternative minority group spaces. For example, Sam discussed his use of crystal methamphetamine and other drugs among gay and lesbian youth as being linked to the desire for 'intense conversations' and their ostracism from the heteronormative 'mainstream':

Yeah with the stimulants it's certainly sensation seeking. If you feel more sensation life feels more meaningful, in a lot of senses because especially for queers and I include bisexuals and gay and lesbians, and trans people – the common dialogues of religion and politics reject them. They don't have a home in mainstream.

There is little research directly attributing substance abuse to rejection from mainstream dialogues and discourses, although Hawkins (2002) explains that alienation from the dominant views of society, low religiosity, and rebelliousness predict greater substance use in adolescence. Thus, bisexual adolescents and young people may turn to more alternative youth subcultures in order to express their sexuality because being bisexual in a heteronormative society may put them on the margins or outside their everyday friendship and support networks at school. Indeed, Cotterell emphasises that 'having friends and being included in the group are among the most important concerns of adolescents' (1994: 259). This was supported by our bisexual adolescent and young adult research participants such as Sam who stated: 'being socially connected is really important to your mental, physical and spiritual health'. Thus, social pressure exists and perhaps is exacerbated within mainstream friendship support networks such as those at school and in local neighbourhoods in relation to those who are bisexual.

However, even if a bisexual young person did feel included and supported in a heterosexual friendship group, these peer groups themselves were also commonly involved in the consumption of alcohol and other substances as these behaviours were signifiers of one's membership of a 'cool' friendship group for many young people regardless of sexuality (Duff 2003). There were some perceived benefits of drug use amongst our research participants which are similar to those expressed by many heterosexual young people (Hatzenbuehler *et al.* 2008). Like many heterosexual young people, Victoria stated that sometimes she did enjoy 'getting pissed', and that drinking was a way to alleviate her shyness with other people in social settings.

The links between exclusion by inclusion of bisexual youth in gay and lesbian communities and substance abuse

Balsam and Mohr (2007) found bisexual young people experience higher levels of identity confusion and lower levels of both self-disclosure and community connection in comparison to their gay and lesbian peers, which may increase isolation, affect self-esteem, and promote risky behaviours. As Victoria explained:

> There's a lot of pressure to kind of conform to certain modes of behaviour [in the gay/lesbian community], or to sort of prove yourself, like prove how gay you are, and if you're bisexual it doesn't really help because people sort of don't trust that as much. So that can lead to just feeling ostracised.

However, although many bisexual young people report a disconnection with the gay/lesbian communities, they tend to feel a similar sense of alienation from the bisexual community, perceiving it as small, invisible, or with little social networking opportunities for young people (Entrup and Firestein 2007). As Mike, a health service provider working with GLBT youth, said in relation to the Australian bisexual scene 'There's no bi nightclubs, or you know, bi bars, or things like that, it's either gay bars or straight bars'.

Isolating oneself from the gay/lesbian and bisexual communities was one of a number of problematic strategies and methods used by bisexual young people to cope with discrimination, marginalisation and feelings of exclusion due to sexuality and/or age. Sam explained that sometimes he would restrict his socialising, not visiting certain places or participating in certain events within non-heterosexual spaces, in order not to be drawn into the culture of substance abuse. Thus, isolation from 'queer spaces' is not only a catalyst for substance abuse for bisexual young people but can also be seen as a protector against it. This is because of what appears to be some sense of normalisation of substance use and risk-taking behaviours amongst gay and lesbian communities within which bisexual young people may try to socialise (Howard and Arcuri 2006; Rosario *et al.* 2004):

> They might become part of the gay community, and because it's bit of a monoculture type of club, so when they do that that's when they get confronted with drugs ... So if they start then going to those clubs, then they'll be confronted with ecstasy users, and then they might come across ecstasy and might experiment.
>
> (Mike, GLBT youth health worker)

Victoria discussed the substance abuse in gay and lesbian 'scenes' where people have a 'pack mentality'. Sam explained that when he went to parties within the 'gay scene' he 'got off his head', but didn't find a sense of belonging there. He also stated that ecstasy may create a sense of intimacy and confidence for bisexual young men within the gay community where they want to express themselves to fellow gay peers but are self-conscious as they could be rejected.

Despite the experiences and perceptions of exclusion and attempts at feeling included by bisexual young people within gay/lesbian communities, these communities can be of positive significance to bisexual young people, particularly in relation to social support needs and mental health issues. GLBT youth worker Mike believed that there are more similarities between the gay/lesbian community and bisexuality than there is with heterosexuality. Victoria also related to the gay and lesbian communities through her friendships. She explained how she easily made friends and came out in her university environment, where 'pretty much everybody was gay or queer of some description', that not many of them drank excessively or took drugs, and that they were 'pretty grounded'.

Exclusion by inclusion of bisexual youth in mainstream and GLBT health services

In their UK study, King and McKeown (2003) found that gay and lesbian participants were more likely to be open about their sexuality to both mainstream and gay/lesbian doctors and mental health professionals than bisexual men and women who would either 'pass' as straight or same-sex attracted. In particular, bisexual women were less likely to report that they had received a positive reaction from mental health professionals. Similarly:

bisexual women and men seek help for sexual orientation issues less frequently and rate their services as less helpful with sexual orientation concerns than gay and lesbian participants ... participants urged providers to validate bisexuality as legitimate and healthy, to be accurately informed about bisexual issues, and to intervene proactively with bisexual clients.

(Page 2004: 139)

Bisexual research participants were more likely to report that clinicians 'invalidated and pathologised' the sexual orientation of the client by either assuming the client's bisexuality 'was connected to clinical issues when the client didn't agree, or assumed that bisexual attractions and behavior would disappear when the client regained psychological health' (Page 2004: 139). The bisexual participants in Dobinson *et al.*'s (2005) research said they did not receive appropriate information about sexual health from health service providers, and indeed, were recipients of inappropriate jokes and comments, voyeurism and pathologisation from these providers. The participants called for the development of bi-specific health and community services for bisexuals as well as better competency and sensitivity training for providers in both gay/lesbian and mainstream services. Some of the bi-specific services they called for included counselling/mental health services, coming out groups, telephone support services, the development of bisexual social spaces, as well as undertaking a large-scale media and public information campaign. Interestingly, Dobinson *et al.*'s (2005) adult participants also called for the establishment of services and programs specifically for bisexual young people, including a helpline, mentoring programs and support groups, which they had found lacking in their own youth.

In our research, there were varied opinions about gay/lesbian and heteronormative health service providers in relation to where bisexual young people could and would go for support in relation to mental health concerns and substance abuse. Mike explained that bisexual people are more likely to get support from a gay and lesbian service as all these services would say they are 'GLBT friendly'. However, he also found that bisexual young people would use mainstream services, particularly if one of their coping strategies was not to disclose their bisexual orientation and/or behaviours. Adolescent and young adult participants in our research such as Michelle said that she would not feel comfortable going to her local general practitioners as she thinks they have 'no clue' on sexual issues. When asked if he would feel comfortable using a new mainstream doctor or service, Sam responded that it would be 'messed up' and 'weird doing that'. Victoria said that in the past she did seek support from a mainstream service which was 'fine about' her sexual orientation, but she believed they were of a poor quality in general. Sarah, a GLBT youth health service provider, said there was no common training for mainstream health providers in relation to sexual diversity, which may cause complexities and concerns in supporting bisexual youth (see Goldfried 2001). She explained that 'a lot of [mainstream] services would be heterocentric in that they don't kind of get the same-sex attraction side of things'.

Conversely, in gay and lesbian oriented services, Mike explained that young bisexual people may 'fall through the gaps', as they may only be asked about their same-sex relationships and behaviours and therefore feel reluctant to disclose their heterosexual relationships and behaviours. This is similar to their experiences in gay/lesbian youth groups as bisexual youth may 'pass' as same-sex attracted as they find that other bisexuals do not frequent these peer groups, which are often organised and attended by gay and lesbian youth. Thus, 'the invisibility and isolation they experience in broader society is mirrored in these youth groups' (Travers and O'Brien 1997: 131). Research with Australian youth in relation to gay/lesbian youth social and support groups found that they were more likely to be exclusively attracted to the same sex and to identify as gay or lesbian (Hillier 2007). Hillier states that same-sex attracted groups provide the 'increase in support and acceptance' that allows previously bisexual-identifying young people 'to acknowledge their [gay and lesbian] attractions more freely and match their identity to them' (2007: 5). While this may certainly be the case for some young people, another probability is not raised within this report: that bisexual young people may feel coerced to *mismatch* their attractions to a gay or lesbian identity in order to gain acceptance and support from this group membership. A young bisexual participant in our research, Bonnie, was a volunteer in a queer youth group who commented: 'I'm always the one putting in my bit about bi stuff, because the guy who runs it is gay and he's very gay. And so he never says anything about bi stuff.'

In relation to bisexual support groups and services, Mike mentioned that in the only renowned bisexual support group in his Australian city, the members were older, and young people are more likely to want to participate in a youth-specific service or group. This may indicate a need for more professional support groups for young bisexual people as well as bi-youth specific social networks.

However, there is some debate in regard to whether sexual categorisation should be either inclusive or specific. Can there be a balance of both, or should umbrella-terms like 'queer' be used (Gammon and Isgro 2006)? How do we acknowledge the specificity of bisexuality but simultaneously step away from putting people into exclusionary divisive sexual categories? It may be beneficial for support services to put less emphasis on categorising people with such terms or resorting to such categories, but at the same time a balance must be achieved in embracing minority-within-minority populations such as the bisexual population. When asked what he would like to see in services supporting young bisexual people's wellbeing, Mike responded with, 'look, just to acknowledge their existence' and demonstrate their inclusion of all GLBT people. They also need to demonstrate their awareness of differences, they are 'distinct from gays and lesbians in the sense of having different health needs, different identity needs and different health issues'.

This supports the findings of Dobinson *et al.* (2005) who recommended visible inclusion of bi-specificity in all public health services as well as public health education including a large-scale media and information campaign. Sarah stated that all health services should adopt more inclusive terms such as 'same-sex attracted' or 'not quite sure' in acknowledging the diversity of sexual orientation, as well as language that is common among youth cultures such as 'not quite straight'. She also suggested that it would be useful for all services to have bi-specific youth policies, programs and practices as well as inclusive resources and programs so that the particular requirements and requests of individual bisexual youth can be catered for.

One final area of problematic health service provision discussed by adolescent and young people in our research was school counsellors and student welfare officers. It appears that counsellors and other adults in school settings could enforce closeting of same-sex attraction or passing as straight in young people. For example, Bonnie told us about her visit to a school counsellor who did not provide her with any immediate resources or direction for her bisexuality. She came out as bisexual soon afterward to her close friends at school and thus received the support of her heterosexual peers without any institutional support from the 'school counsellor'. Another adolescent, Andrea, came out as bisexual in a school that was proud of its reputation for having clear anti-homophobic student welfare policies and health education resources. Yet, even in that environment, she found that her refusal to label her sexuality as lesbian made her feel alien:

> It's like they can only do all this good stuff for you if you fit in to the boxes. So okay, they've got more boxes than most schools, but they're still boxes. ... your name tag has to read, 'hi, I'm gay' or 'hi, I'm lesbian', so they can go to their sex kits and pull out the words, the program, and all that school stuff that are for people like you. ... I did crack it one day when the counsellor kept pushing me to say what I was, and I went, 'Look, if I have to wear a sticky label, I'm a UFO, an unidentified fucking object'. I got detention for that and all these warnings about being promiscuous, STDs, the lot. They kinda went into a panic ... The thing is, I wasn't even having full-on sex with anyone but I was feeling shitty about their boxy ways, and I let them have it with the UFO thing. I was quite proud of my creative imagery. You'd think my English teacher would be pleased, but he said I was disrespectful. That's what he called it. Well, how about respecting me in letting me tell you what my sexuality is or isn't?

Conclusion: inclusion with specificity

As our discussion of the available literature and our own research illustrates, mainstream and GLBT health research, resources and service providers, and the broader heterosexual and gay/lesbian communities need to acknowledge the complexities bisexual young people need to address such as invisibility or omission within a sexual dichotomy, not having a strong identity as a collective group, and the discrimination, isolation and marginalisation that exists from both heterosexual and homosexual communities. We therefore propose an 'inclusion with specificity' model, whereby specific acknowledgement and understanding of bisexual people as a group takes place. At the same time, the external imposition of categories and labels should be limited, and the individual's self-ascription and agency in how they see and label themselves, and the kinds of specific and/or inclusive services they wish to use, are available.

As adult health researchers, health providers and health educators working within queer and mainstream communities, we need to ask how health research, policies, programs and practices reflect the dominant or residual discourses of hierarchical sexual dualisms. These may be increasingly out of step with the emergent shifting contexts and diverse sexual cultures that today's young people are immersed within, engaging with, and negotiating (Savin-Williams 2005).

In conclusion, this engagement with sexual multiplicity rather than compressing it into duality, and making visible bisexuality rather than submerging it into heterosexual or homosexual homogenising categories, will ultimately be transformative in creating individual, social and institutional healthy systems and cultures. This will take our young 'X-files' into a healthy future wherein, as adults themselves, they will continue the work toward sex-gender justice. As both young bisexual participants and adult health service providers have shown in our research, bisexual young people are part of the process of transferring internalised distress over 'messing up sex files' to the external bodies, discourses and 'filing systems' that have constructed those exclusionary and dichotomising files in the first place. In order that sexualities, relationships and educational and health services may more effectively acknowledge that 'desire is multi-faceted, contradictory, subversive: its inevitable social organisation requires that we are engaged in a continuous conversation about both its possibilities and limits' (Weeks 1995: 50).

2.13 Hope of a nation – experiences of social exclusion giving rise to spaces of inclusion for people living with HIV and AIDS in South Africa: a reflection

Greer Lamaro

Introduction

South Africa is a country of diversities, contrasts and contradictions; it boasts eleven official languages in addition to countless tribal dialects, a rich diversity of racial and cultural groups, and a landscape encompassing everything from tranquil beaches to rugged bush lands and rocky mountains. South Africa also has one of the highest rates of HIV/AIDS in the world. No one particular group is affected by the virus – rather, it is indiscriminate. Similarly, responses to HIV are diverse, and can be starkly contradictory. This author lived among the Xhosa people in rural Eastern Cape, working in community development. The program was a population-based youth empowerment program around HIV prevention. The work involved engaging youth in a range of civic participation activities, and networking with other community based groups and organisations, health and social services, and government departments. Here, the author reflects upon her experience, drawing out a narrative of the lived experiences of social exclusion and social connectedness for people living with HIV/AIDS in rural Eastern Cape.

The reflection will draw out the paradox of how the high prevalence of stigma and discrimination towards those with the illness, and their subsequent experience of social exclusion, actually creates opportunities for social connectedness through support group participation. This in turn is fashioning an emerging social movement breaking down barriers of stigma, and contributing to broader social change to support HIV action in this diverse and sometimes contradictory social environment.

The reflection begins by outlining the current context and underlying determinants of the proliferation of HIV in the Eastern Cape, including a discussion of exclusion as a determinant. An exploration of how exclusion is also experienced as an outcome of positive HIV status follows. An explanation of how the experience of exclusion can be transformed into spaces of connectedness, and implications for health promotion practice in this context, will be presented.

The context – contemporary rural South Africa

South Africa has one of the most prolific HIV/AIDS epidemics in the world. The projected prevalence rates are that one in three women aged fifteen to thirty years, and one in four men of the same age group, will be infected by 2015 (Iliffe 2006). South Africa is not unique or alone in this. Indeed, much of Africa – in particular Sub-Saharan Africa – is experiencing high infection rates, along with Latin America, Asia and increasingly the Middle East. What is unique about the South African situation is the indiscriminate nature of the illness. The epidemic in South Africa is not predominantly prevalent in any one particular sub-group, but rather all groups are affected (Iliffe 2006). However, for a variety of structural and cultural reasons, certain groups are more vulnerable, including women and the majority black population (Zungu-Dirwayi *et al.* 2007).

The underlying determinants of the epidemic in South Africa are multiple and varied, being structural, political, systemic, cultural and environmental in nature. It is beyond the scope of this chapter to address them all. However, a few key notions will be discussed, particularly the link between the transitional nature of contemporary South Africa and social exclusion interacting as determinants (Box 2.1).

Transition and exclusion as determinants of HIV

The link between the youths' penchant for pop music and the HIV/AIDS epidemic (as described in Box 2.1) may seem remote at first. However, the two

---

Box 2.1 The changing face of rural South Africa

Gathering at the river to do the washing is more than just undertaking a daily household chore for young girls in rural communities around the Eastern Cape. It is a social gathering. A task that is already laborious in time is stretched out even longer as the girls take the opportunity to laugh, sing and chat together. It is an opportunity for social gathering and connecting, as it was for their *mamas* and *makhulus* (grandmothers) before them. It is a time honoured and favoured pastime in their traditional lives. Only a few things have changed. Rather than hearing traditional Xhosa gospel songs being sung, you're likely to hear Beyonce's latest chart topper being belted out. The girls call to each other not by their traditional Xhosa names, but rather, using their adopted western names of Whitney or Ivy, introduced to them through popular American soap operas. Then one receives a text message on her cellular phone from her boyfriend – he wants her to go to the road to meet him. She can't. She has to finish washing the clothes by hand, and then collect wood for the fire to cook the bread for supper tonight.

are really not that far removed from each other. What this scene represents is the transitional context of South Africa today, particularly as it is experienced by young people. Youth are living with disparate cognitive information from their traditional cultures and increasingly from Western cultures. South Africa has been described as '... the exemplar of African modernity' (van der Westhuizen 2008: 45), as it seeks to establish a unique and contemporary national identity in an increasingly globalised setting. Exposure to multiple cultural inputs, traditional and new, makes the task complex, as South Africa mediates between notions of *Africanism* vs. *Eurocentrism*;

> Africanism and eurocentrism are the two rallying concepts for an ongoing dialectic that may characterise political and cultural discourse in South Africa for decades to come. There is an impatient quest for a synthesis of these two positions from both sides. As yet, the struggle to install one version over the other as common sense is an ongoing one and no synthesis is in sight.
>
> (Schutte 2000: 218)

Added to this is the complexity of identifying within the broader 'African' identity. Often, Africa is conceived as a homogenous entity (Crewe 2002) rather than the rich tapestry of diversities it is; a tapestry that is dynamic and constantly evolving (Yewah 2008).

For youth in rural parts of South Africa, this context contributes to difficulties in rationalising their future aspirations with the reality of their daily lives in traditional communities. It is a context in which everybody has a cellular phone, yet few have access to employment or finances to sustain adequate basic living standards. There is comprehensive cellular phone coverage, yet inadequately covered roads, pit latrines and dwellings. This interfacing of the traditional with the modern has implications creating conditions of exclusion for rural youth in the Eastern Cape, and the subsequent proliferation of HIV and AIDS in these areas.

Notions of social exclusion permeate discourses of HIV as both a determinant and an outcome. Evidence suggests that social exclusion may be one of multiple factors contributing to the development of the HIV epidemic (Zungu-Dirwayi *et al.* 2007). People in predominantly Xhosa rural areas of the Eastern Cape experience multiple forms of exclusion on the basis of race, class, gender, location and socio-economic status (Zungu-Dirwayi *et al.* 2007). Many of these factors are inter-connected, and have compounding effects for exclusion (Lee *et al.* 2002). In turn, their experience of exclusion based on these characteristics contributes to a greater vulnerability to HIV (Richter 2001; Parker and Aggleton 2003; Jones 2005).

Youth in traditional rural communities are often excluded from viable education and job opportunities, given their geographical and socio-economic status. While South Africa increasingly participates in global market economies, the capacity to do so, and the benefits of doing such are unequally distributed throughout the country. For a range of interacting structural and socio-cultural reasons, rural communities are greatly disadvantaged and experience great poverty and few education and employment opportunities. Youth in these areas would often lament the lack of opportunities to find jobs, pursue professional careers or undertake entrepreneurial ventures. They would often speak in terms of 'otherness', the 'others' being the wealthy white population and the burgeoning urban black bourgeois. This has implications for the spread of HIV among the isolated and poor rural youth, as it has been found that those who are financially excluded are more likely to contract AIDS than those with greater financial resources (Zungu-Dirwayi *et al.* 2007).

Rural youth are also excluded from access to health information and services. While the cultural evolution occurs across the nation, advances in technology, information dissemination, and other key structures and resources largely lag behind in the low income rural areas. People excluded from access to health information also experience higher infection rates (Zungu-Durwayi *et al.* 2007). An example highlighting unreliable health information dissemination occurred during 2007 when a brand of condoms was recalled nationwide due to a manufacturing fault. This information progressed like a game of 'Chinese Whispers' through rural communities, going something along the following lines:

Manufacturing fault and subsequent recall

↓

'This batch is faulty'

↓

'These condoms are not good enough to protect you from HIV, so should not be used'

↓

'Condoms cause HIV, so should not be used'.

It is conceivable that a combination of factors contributed to the eventuality of this situation, including language and cultural barriers. However, it also demonstrates the inadequacy of reliable health information and services in rural Eastern Cape areas. A combination of structural, economic and cultural factors interacts to create this dynamic.

Similarly, myth and misunderstanding further contribute to the HIV epidemic in the Eastern Cape. Commonly cited beliefs are that HIV results from *ubugqwirha* (witchcraft); that a man can be cured by having sexual intercourse with a virgin girl; or that condoms are a Western-derived conspiracy to spread HIV among black people. Research in other communities also authenticates the role of myth and misunderstanding as barriers to preventing HIV (Birdsall and Kelly 2005). The interplay of several factors in the propagation of myth and misunderstanding is evident. For instance, limited access to correct health information in rural areas, owing to a range of cultural and structural factors, contributes to the propagation of misleading information in these communities.

Gender based exclusion is another key determinant in the spread of HIV, and is also complicated by the transitional nature of society. Significant culturally-based gender inequalities exist in South Africa, stemming from traditional gender roles. Women are subject to greater disadvantage than their male counterparts (Fassin and Schneider 2003; Ballard *et al.* 2005; Campbell *et al.* 2006; Cuhna 2007). Subsequently, women are commonly excluded from a range of vital opportunities, including access to financial independence, education and decision making in relationships. Polygamy is common, in part owing to traditional associations of status for men being associated with many female partners (Alexander and Uys 2002; Skinner and Mfecane 2004). Consequently, women are generally disempowered to exercise power or decision making in their relationships, including decisions about their own sexual health practices. Women are generally not empowered to refuse sexual relations with their husbands or insist on the use of condoms, for fear of violent retribution. Thus, gender based vulnerability to HIV is a stark reality for many women, and becomes poignant when hearing the women's stories. One woman explained how her husband must go to the city to work. When he calls her, she must go and join him, despite heavy commitments of caring for six children (including two infants), agriculture and tending cattle. She states that she is aware he probably has multiple sexual partners in the city and thus may have contracted HIV, but feels she can neither confront him about it nor refuse his demands. She revealed how every time she coughs or has any kind of small pain, she fears it could be HIV.

However, with the changing face of South Africa, young people are becoming increasingly aware and active around matters of citizenship and rights, including gender equality, although vast chasms exist in communication between generation. Young people find it extremely difficult to talk to older people about issues of gender, sexuality and HIV. Campbell and colleagues (2006: 133) state that 'Many parents simply refuse to acknowledge the very possibility of youth sexuality' and 'certainly never discuss sex with their children'. Thus, they conclude that young people are being excluded from respect and recognition in society. This was also found to be the case in rural Eastern Cape communities by this author and colleagues, through interactions with youth who communicated that:

'In more traditional areas the older generation seems to be against young people having relationships, so they have to keep it behind closed doors. So it's almost an oppressive effect of not being able to talk to their families freely.'

'There's no real chance to talk over contraception or about the relationship.'

'the older generation and mothers not talking openly about relationships – it's stopping them from learning how to negotiate sex. Here ... it's all very hidden ... you don't even see couples holding hands out here.'

Inherent in the exclusionary divide between generations is once again the transient nature of contemporary South Africa as experienced by youth, interacting with traditional normative processes.

Du Toit (2004: 999) notes that social exclusion could be conceived as 'one moment or component in complex and multileveled processes of deprivation'. Similarly, de Haan (1998) considers social exclusion to function as a result of multiple processes of discrimination and exclusion, rather than a state affecting a particular population of outcasts or outsiders (such as South African youth existing within the traditional and the transitional). The above discussion intended to highlight the interplay of some key structural and cultural factors that interconnect, allowing exclusion circumstances to prevail and contribute to the proliferation of HIV in rural Eastern Cape. The focus will now to turn to social exclusion as an outcome of HIV for those living with the virus.

The role of stigma and discrimination in the experience of exclusion as an outcome

In addition to being a key determinant of HIV, social exclusion is also experienced as an outcome for people living with HIV and AIDS. PWHA experience exclusion in many facets of daily life, including exclusion from social networks, civic participation, and access to health and social resources. This exclusion may occur for multiple reasons, including deteriorating health and a physical inability to participate in civic society, socioeconomic barriers (including poverty due poor health limiting one's capacity to work), structural or systemic barriers (like poor availability of and access to health, social and welfare systems, and limited treatment options) and stigma and discrimination. It is exclusion due to stigma and discrimination that will be the focus here.

People's lived experiences of the epidemic are affected by how individuals, the community and the nation respond. Responses in South Africa have proliferated and diversified over recent years (Birdsall and Kelly 2005; Jewkes 2006). These responses are affected by a combination of socio-cultural factors including class, race, gender and competing discourses, including medical, political and religious (Kauffman and Lindauer 2004; Squire 2007), reflecting the diverse context of South Africa. However, to date, responses of individuals and communities have often been typified by high levels of stigma and discrimination towards HIV and AIDS, and PWHA. Several factors have been identified as drivers of HIV related stigma in South Africa, including a deep-seated culture of fear, poor availability of legitimate health information, limited social opportunities for dialogue and communication, negative connotations associated with notions of poverty and moralities, and a desire to create 'otherness', among many others (Petros *et al.* 2006; Campbell *et al.* 2007).

The implications of stigma for social exclusion are great, and can be devastating for those affected. Exclusion is commonly experienced by PWHA through decreased social status and downward social mobility (Mills 2006), and being shunned by the community. A common attitude among some sections of the community towards PWHA is that they (PWHA) 'are just silly', with reference to their sexual behaviour, and there is a tendency to victim-blame. Such attitudes and tendencies are imbedded in a moral discourse and a desire by the excluders to create an 'otherness' of these perceived deviates (Mills 2006; Petros *et al.* 2006). (For further examination of othering and exclusion see Chapter 2.14, Othering, marginalisation and pathways to exclusion and health, by Barter-Godfrey and Taket.)

So great are the effects of stigma, discrimination and subsequent exclusion, that people are reluctant to access vital services. This is evident by the low rates of people undergoing voluntary counselling and testing (VCT) (Hutchinson and Mahlalela 2006). Simply being seen to be entering a room at the local clinic where VCT may be conducted is enough to pass a social death sentence (Day *et al.* 2003). Coupled with this, particularly in rural areas, is the fear of lack of confidentiality. Many community members are emphatic that they would not test for HIV as they feel that clinic staff would gossip about their health status with others in the community. The concept of confidentiality is understood; it is just not a concept in which locals place great surety. These fears may be legitimate given study findings that confidentiality breaches were a possible occurrence in rural communities in the Eastern Cape (Hutchinson and Mahlalela 2006).

Consequently, people often travel to other communities to undergo VCT. For those who lack the resources or ability to travel, a process of self-exclusion from accessing and participating in health services is common, in order to avoid the anticipated greater consequences of exclusion by the community. Similar occurrences have been found in other South African communities also (Daftary *et al.* 2007).

For those who do undergo VCT, it does not necessarily follow that they then disclose their status or access local health and social services, like medical treatment or support groups. Rather, many feel the need to hide their positive status for fear of social stigmatisation and exclusion. Local HIV support groups do exist, but as with VCT, have been widely under-utilised. As with accessing VCT, to be seen attending a support group meeting is sometimes enough to bring stigma and exclusion from community members. Exclusion (including self-exclusion) from accessing health and social services can have serious negative implications for the health and wellbeing of PWHA.

Despite this, in order for the support groups to continue to operate, there exist brave people who are willing to face fear and discrimination in order to participate. For these people, the personal and social gains from inclusion within the group outweigh the negative consequences. What must be considered about those who do participate is that they are possibly somewhat less excluded than those who do not attend. That is, commonly they are people who have some capacity to access resources to enable participation (e.g. finances, transport, information and social networks). For instance, regular meetings of one particular support group at a hospital were mostly attended by women who were family or friends of hospital staff, or had been receiving medical treatment at the hospital. Thus, they already had access to resources to attend the clinic or access to social channels and health information to become aware of the support group. These are the PWHA on the margins of society who are able to be reached and who are able to connect. The challenge is reaching and engaging those who are beyond the margins. This includes those already weakened and incapacitated by sickness, out-of-school youth and young single mothers. These groups often experience the compounding effects of multiple exclusions arising from various categories of otherness, and make it very difficult for these people to connect to communities.

The changing face of South Africa revisited

However, reflecting the dynamic nature of South African society, responses to HIV in South Africa are both increasing and diversifying (Birdsall and Kelly 2005; Jewkes 2006). In particular, community-led initiatives have proliferated.

HIV support groups are one type of community-led intervention that has developed. The profile and role of HIV support groups continues to expand throughout the Eastern Cape, involving PWHA, local health care workers, support group advocates, community based organisations (CBOs), non-governmental organisations (NGOs), and increasingly, faith based organisations (FBOs) (Birdsall and Kelly 2005). Support groups in the area now often go beyond the traditional role of such groups, expanding their activities and target audience. Their proliferation and mobilisation is developing into a social movement, promoting connectedness of PWHA. Definitions of social movements abound. It is beyond the scope of this chapter to critique them; however Ballard and colleagues (2005: 617) examine various explanations, before deriving their own. They contend social movements are 'politically and/or socially directed collectives, often involving multiple organisations and networks, focused on changing one or more elements of the social, political and economic system within which they are located'. The activities of the support group network operating in the Eastern Cape provide a good example. For instance, from humble beginnings of meeting to talk about issues around HIV, including experiences of social exclusion, a range of activities is now undertaken that goes beyond social support, and connects the groups with the wider community. Regular community awareness days are a major initiative and have become a predominant strategy in trying to break down stigma and discrimination and promote greater connectedness for PWHA. These events include the provision of accurate information about HIV contagion and prevention, and provide VCT services. These days aim to break down stigma and discrimination arising from fear, myth and misinformation about the virus. The days put a human face to HIV, by giving members of the community of PWHA a voice by disclosing their status and advocating on behalf of PWHA. They show PWHA as ordinary community members, professionals, faithful wives and mothers, and thus break down barriers around 'otherness', derived from perceptions of immorality and sexual deviance by PWHA that transgress social norms. Culturally valued methods of communication and expression are utilised, like drama and song, to disseminate information in a manner that is legitimate and appropriate. In doing so, PWHA are able to reach out to and engage other community members through media that are common to and valued by community members – both with HIV and those without – thus finding commonalities and a metaphorical place of connectedness in culture. The organisation and running of the events involves collaboration between the local-based support groups, community groups (like cultural performance groups), community leaders and committees, hospital and clinic staff, local government officials, and representatives of other NGOs, CBOs and FBOs, thus providing opportunities for PWHA and members of the wider community to engage with key stakeholders.

In addition, advocacy activities are undertaken by support groups to promote inclusion and connectedness, further lending to an emerging social movement. Support groups are key drivers in political campaigns around HIV issues, including pushing for official recognition by the government of the link between HIV and AIDS, and access to antiretroviral drugs for PWHA. Local support groups work in partnership with other organisations and NGOs to raise issues on political and social agendas, and have become key agents influencing government action around HIV and AIDS issues over recent years. This collaborative social action has contributed to 'a time when the many voices of people infected and affected by HIV in the country were starting to gain a hearing' (Squire 2007: 4).

Other activities undertaken by support groups include establishing income generating projects like agricultural or textile projects. These projects link participants with local government and other key stakeholders at various levels, building their capacity to participate in civic and bureaucratic processes (for instance, through fundraising). Participants develop skills and capacities for employment and income generation, whilst providing necessary goods for consumption, and thus revealing an avenue for connection with society via participation in markets. This linking on vertical and horizontal planes helps to promote the capacity of PWHA to 'live positively' as an active member of the community, and develop commonalities to form linking bonds between them and other community members.

Thus, in reflecting upon the role of HIV support groups in the Eastern Cape, several elements of a social movement are evident. Support groups have expanded their scope to advocate for and address issues of equity and social justice for PWHA. They are working to address and effect change in social, physical and economic environments for greater inclusion of PWHA. They are acting as agents of empowerment for PWHA by creating environments and opportunities for civic participation by PWHA, linking PWHA with members of the broader society in which they live, and engaging a range of stakeholders at various levels in the process. HIV support groups and their members are gaining strength as individuals and units, and developing their capacities to undertake necessary community development and social change activities effectively.

Continuing to move forward: implications for health promotion

HIV and AIDS in South Africa is a complex issue, arising from a multitude of determinants, and having an array of impacts. It is necessary, therefore, that interventions to reduce the impact of HIV on communities be diverse and comprehensive.

Strategies need to be aimed at both HIV prevention and management. Both can be addressed through a social exclusion/inclusion lens. Preventive action needs to go beyond a simple model of HIV information provision. Issues of social stigma, discrimination and exclusion need to be targeted in order to address the root causes currently acting as barriers to equity and social justice, and contributing to vulnerabilities to HIV. Given the implications of stigma for the proliferation and maintenance of the HIV epidemic, interventions focused on addressing stigma are necessary. This is supported by Skinner and Mfecane (2004) who argue that all interventions to address HIV should address the multiple forms of stigma endemic in South Africa and implicated in the HIV epidemic. This would involve developing a better understanding of the nature of stigma and its causes (such as those identified by Campbell *et al.* 2007) and addressing them from a determinant's perspective. This may involve the creation of opportunities for dialogue around issues of HIV (like determinants of HIV and HIV related stigma), and enhanced community based empowerment interventions around issues including gender and race. Exactly *how* to do this effectively should be the focus of further research.

Interventions promoting social inclusion of PWHA also need to be considered for the management of the epidemic. In doing so, Campbell and colleagues (2006) contend that interventions needs shift from a top-down model, toward a decentralised, community-led model. Such interventions should focus on the broader socio-cultural factors implicated in experiences of HIV, including stigma and social exclusion, and recognise the ability to empower people by connecting them with each other. Ways of doing this are broad and limited only by the imagination. Support groups in the Eastern Cape provide a good example of local, grass roots action to address HIV prevention and management by addressing issues of stigma and barriers to inclusion for PWHA.

However, in working to ensure cultural appropriateness and local empowerment, initiatives must be careful not to exclude other external players. Rather, there should be a focus on developing locally led initiatives, whilst still engaging 'outsiders' and 'others' as learners and participants. Notable among community development projects throughout the Eastern Cape is the high level of volunteerism from local, indigenous community members. A number of international volunteers are involved, and a small number of volunteers of other South African races are evident – though many have lived or worked among the communities for a substantial time. Promoting greater volunteerism among people external to rural Eastern Cape communities could go some way to breaking down racially based conceptions of HIV, in a country that has been described as 'racially insecure and still racially raw' (Crewe 2002: 451), and in which HIV/AIDS is often considered and addressed as a ' "black" plague' (Alexander and Uys 2002: 300). Crewe (2002) contends that unless racism is challenged, HIV responses will continue to develop within a racially based framework, rather than addressing the need for social change in this area. Furthermore, Crewe (2002: 453) posits that the South African HIV epidemic provides a 'new lens to look at ... old issues that have to be addressed'. Connecting traditional and rural communities with broader South Africa through volunteerism may be a mechanism to separate notions of race from the HIV epidemic, and address key social determinants of HIV proliferation in South Africa. However, the challenge of *how* to do this against such a political and transitional backdrop (a situation described by Kelly and Van Vlaenderen [1996: 1236] as one in which people have been 'deeply committed to political struggle rather than co-operation') remains. It certainly warrants the dedication of time and research to investigate mechanisms through which a social environment characterised by trust and solidarity can be developed, and co-operative participation promoted and achieved.

The contribution of local interventions to the effort to conquer HIV cannot be discounted (Foster 2004 in Birdsall and Kelly 2005). Tackling the HIV epidemic in South Africa requires a cohesive approach, involving players from all sectors of society. This is the hope *for* a nation – that in this post-apartheid era, cohesive responses to HIV can be developed that do not subscribe to racial, class, socio-economic or other socially subscribed boundaries. Only in this way can we realise the hope *of* a nation – a united one, free from the social burden of HIV and the associated stigma.

The example of HIV support groups in the Eastern Cape is a fine example of how adversity can be turned into opportunity. From experiences of exclusion, people involved can find a space and place for connection and opportunities for broader social inclusion. Alexander and Uys (2002) argue that to address HIV in South Africa, a conceptual shift is needed away from focusing on what makes people susceptible to HIV/AIDS (which they contend has resulted in misdirected and failed responses to date), towards emphasising the positive factors and experiences that can be built upon. HIV support groups in the Eastern Cape not only provide a good opportunity to do this in order to address HIV, but also for addressing broader issues of exclusion and connectedness. The mechanisms that have allowed Eastern Cape HIV support groups to function and flourish need to be better understood and work around social connectedness for marginalised people and communities. Support for such groups and their work needs to continue from local community members and the wider community of practitioners, researchers and key stakeholders alike.

Having said that, I would like to acknowledge the work of Transcape NPO, and all those community members and health workers actively engaged with HIV support groups in the Eastern Cape. Nithabatha xaxheba no nika ilizwa – *umntu nugmntu ngabantu.* Siyabulela kakhulu. (Thank you for your willingness to participate and give voice. *A person is a person only through other people* – a Xhosa proverb emphasising humanity).

Also and especially, to Maureen Lamaro – my inspiration, encouragement, and motivation – 'It was the best and the worst'.

2.14 Othering, marginalisation and pathways to exclusion in health

Sarah Barter-Godfrey and Ann Taket

Introduction

An important part of our understanding of social exclusion is that, rather than a dichotomy of included or excluded, there is recognition of long-term processes, grounded in social dynamics and individual experiences. One of these processes is 'othering': marginalisation through being 'the other'. This chapter explores othering and illustrates how it can operate it multiple ways with both positive and negative effects (and indeed affects), acting as an inclusionary process in some circumstances and an exclusionary one in other circumstances. We explore othering in both inter- and intra-personal terms.

We begin by offering a brief overview of the concept of othering, and the related notion of stigma. The process of othering is then explored in a number of different ways. First of all we examine how stigma, secrets and dissociation act as exclusionary othering processes for victims of abuse. We then turn to look at othering and the self in health protective decision-making, exploring how candidacy acts as an inclusionary process in breast screening. The final section explores some more general implications in terms of othering, health, and inclusive health care practices.

Othering and stigma

Othering is the social, linguistic and psychological mechanism that distinguishes 'us' from 'them', the normal from the deviant (Johnson et al. 2004; Grove and Zwi 2006). Othering marks and names the other, providing a definition of their otherness, which in turn creates social distance, and marginalises, dis-empowers and excludes (Weis 1995). Some have argued that othering serves a psychological purpose, where an 'exclusionary urge' (Hubbard 1998: 281) satisfies a need to keep psycho- and socio-spatial proximity 'clean' from deviant, dirty or threatening others, and maintain moral normality. Freud (1930) suggested that othering was an inevitable narcissism; that peaceful groups are made possible only by the presence of others that could be viewed negatively. Ideas of 'in-group' and 'out-group' were illuminated and explored in the models of Social Identity Theory (Tajfel and Turner 1986).

Reflecting the key principles of othering, Social Identity Theory posits that people are aware of, recognise and evaluate others in terms of adherence or belonging to social groups. This is dependent on *naming the other* to form ideas of group membership; *defining otherness* to identify some people as an in-group and others as an out-group; and *marking the other* so that the out-group members are less favoured when compared to the in-group. In-group differences from the out-group are magnified (increasing social distance) whereas differences within the out-group are minimised (marginalising individuals) and this out-group homogeneity is expressed through negative stereotypes of the group members (Brown 2000). In this way, othering leads to 'in-group identity and out-group antipathy' (Huddy 2007: 130). However, othering is not necessarily the end of the process.

Othering is a key part of the production of stigma. Stigma, literally meaning 'mark', was first described as a social phenomenon in terms of being a 'deeply discrediting' attribute (Goffman 1963: 3). Present conceptualisation of stigma tends to focus on the process and socially constructed devaluation of 'marked' individuals, and the subsequent exclusion from 'unmarked' society. This process is underpinned by othering. Stigma occurs through a categorising label on the basis of an individual attribute (the mark), the marked are separated from the unmarked and the marked label is given meaning by a stereotype, which bears emotional weight and social distance, and excludes the marked through loss of status, and loss or lack of structural power (Link and Phelan 2001b, 2006; Link *et al.* 2004). Stereotypes are collectively understood, through shared cultural knowledge, and can therefore act as 'cues' to an individual that identifies with the marked label, threatening to devalue their identity. In this way, cultural knowledge of the stigmatised can act as form of social control (Bourdieu 1977b) and legitimise exclusionary processes: in this way stigma can be 'highly pragmatic, even tactical' (Yang *et al.* 2007: 1528). Othering represents one of the 'generic processes' of the reproduction of inequality, leading to oppression through identifying 'difference as deficit', the exertion of power through moral identities of superiority or success, and the defensive othering by marginalised people as a means to reassert a credible self (Schwalbe *et al.* 2000: 432). Further inequality processes include subordinate adaptation, elitism of cultural capital, violence and threats, scripting emotional responses and conditioning discourse; maintaining or expanding the gap between the powerful, advantaged, in-groups and the marginalised, disadvantaged others (Schwalbe *et al.* 2000).

Othering, marginalisation, stigma and inequality are inter-related concepts, with a shared component of rewards for being 'normal' or like 'us'; and costs for being different, deviant or like 'them'. For public health issues, these abstract concepts are seen at work in how people respond to health threats. Othering can be a coping mechanism to manage threats to your wellbeing; keeping secrets and non-disclosure are ways of avoiding health threats and being 'othered', as illustrated in the previous chapter around HIV stigma. Conversely, using othering to distinguish yourself from health threats can maintain in-group benefits.

Othering and the self in sexual and domestic violence: how stigma, secrets and dissociation act as exclusionary othering processes for victims of abuse

Secrecy can be a way to avoid being 'marked', to avoid othering, labelling and stigma; secrets are kept to protect self-identity and esteem and out of fear of the consequences of revelation (Afifi and Caughlin 2006). However, keeping secrets, particularly those with 'identity salience' or attributes that make up essential life roles or status, can have negative consequences in itself. The burden of keeping a secret can lead to emotional distress, worry and a lack of self-authenticity. The weight of this burden is inferred from the sense of relief that can be experienced when the secret is shared, but the quality of the relief is dependent on who the secret is revealed to, their reaction, the potential for consequences of revelation and the social and psychological meaning of the secret (Bouman 2003). In some circumstances, the value of keeping a secret outweighs the burden of keeping it, and secrecy can be a coping mechanism for those in fearful situations, such as the threat or experience of sexual and domestic violence.

Secrecy is concomitant with childhood sexual abuse and children may keep abuse secret in order to protect themselves and others from an abuser that threatens further harm for revealing the abuse; secrecy can be a coping mechanism and a containment of abuse (Lyon 1996). It can also be a containment of the consequences of abuse. Denying domestic violence can be a way of avoiding reprisals from the abuser, avoiding police involvement and loss or incarceration of the partner and/or the children's parent, avoiding social worker involvement and fear of losing children into the care system, avoiding losing family support, and avoiding the stigma attached to not being believed. An understanding of what would happen to the 'me', if I became another me that revealed the abuse, and all of the consequences that 'other' me would have to endure can be a strong motivator for secrecy as a coping strategy. Children who have been abused, and do start to reveal that abuse, often tell their secrets gradually, disclosing one aspect of abuse whilst keeping others secret, testing the reaction before further disclosure. In this way, they can bridge the identities of the 'me' who kept the secret and the 'other me' who 'told' (Hershkowitz et al. 2007). 'Not telling' can also be a function of psychological secrecy. Enforced secrecy can inhibit memory formation and full cognition of the abuse, removing the words, labels and naming of abuse needed to encode the story of experiences (Fish and Scott 1999). Here secrecy can represent a form of self-othering, where negative experiences or chaotic thoughts are contained within a second (dissociated) self, to protect the everyday self from feeling, thinking about or remembering traumatic events. This suggests a complex relationship between self and identity, and the need to keep secrets from the self as coping mechanisms to keep a functional self intact.

Creating a 'not-I' compartmentalises trauma within one fragment of the self, and within the social and psychiatric context of Western bio-medical models, the 'experience of "not-I-ness" has become the psychiatric category of Dissociative Identity Disorder' (Scott 1999: 444). For the individual, the trauma is inscribed on the self twice; as the traumatised identity holding the traumatic events within the self-fragments and as the destabilising experience of not-I-ness with emergent psychiatric disorders (Scott 1999).

Self-othering does not have to be necessarily secretive, nor pathological. Jung (1961) referred to having two selves as part of healthy psychological functioning; personality number one is normal and everyday; personality number two is naturalistic and closer to dreaming. Self-othering also emerges in the grey area where your situation is neither imminently harmful nor coherently healthy. For example, sex workers and strippers who use outward 'personas' when working (self othering and keeping part of the self secret from others) and who differentiate themselves from other sex workers (out-group othering) to cope with the realities of their work as well as their stigmatised group identity (Barton 2007). Here, there is secrecy *of* the self and distance from others, but not secrecy *from* the self.

Keeping part of the self secret from the self (e.g. dissociation), self-othering (e.g. sex worker personas) and secrecy (e.g. non-disclosure) represent a range of reactions and coping strategies that may be employed to manage the experience, knowledge and repercussions from sexual abuse, invasion and violence. These processes lead to a marginalisation of the self, marginalised from the self and from others. However, there is a further, malevolent dimension to marginalisation in sexual and domestic violence – that of the intentional marginalisation perpetrated by the abuser. Isolation from peers and family that often occurs with the escalation of domestic violence is marginalising, eroding the victim's connections with their in-group and othering the victim from 'safe' society. Humiliation, a common feature of power and control abuses, is closely related to stigma by making the victim feel 'marked' and discredited (Karlsson 2007). Othering processes that are imposed from without (by the abuser) combined with coping self-othering from within (by the victim), can help to illuminate the complex, threatened and excluded identities of victims of sexual and domestic violence and those victims accessing health and help services, disclosing or keeping secret their experiences.

Othering and the self in health protective decision-making: how candidacy acts as an inclusionary process in breast screening

Candidacy is the notion of who is a good or likely candidate for a disease, and reflects an informal or lay nosology of diseases, health and who is at risk (Taket and Barter-Godfrey 2005). This can be an anthropomorphic characterisation of a disease – he is a heart attack waiting to happen – as an articulation of risk factors and aetiology (Emslie *et al.* 2001).

Conceptualising candidacy as an othering process, we can see that the mark or label is the disease; the stereotype is the lay understanding of causes and occurrences of that disease; and the distance between others is how individually we separate or align ourselves with candidacy. In short, candidacy is othering on the basis of whether that disease happens to 'people like me' and whether my health identity is 'marked' or threatened by that particular disease. Understanding our own candidacy expresses our perceptions of risk burdens and our vulnerability to diseases (Pfeffer 2004).

From an othering perspective, role models are aspirational others, a champion or leader for a desirable in-group. In public health, role modelling is used in health promotion campaigns, with role models acting as the 'face' or 'ambassador', through celebrity or athlete endorsements. Similarly, 'success stories' in weight loss programs use role modelling to encourage identification with the 'common man': if I can do it, so can you. These approaches to health education draw on principles of candidacy by embodying health issues and principles of othering by 'marking' or labelling a person, defining and defined by a culturally understood attribute. Health, diseases and health behaviours become written on the identity of the role model. In response to this positive other, people can identify with and aspire to healthy decisions and behaviours. This continues into health educational materials – can the reader identify with the case studies and illustrations used in information and pamphlets? For breast screening it has been noted that diagrams used to explain self-exam and mammography procedures are unrealistic, with small, perky breasts that bear little resemblance to the post-menopausal bodies of breast screening service-users. The materials, which are supposed to inform and assist women to prepare for mammography, do not identify with the lived experiences of the readers, and create social distance between the service-users and representation of who the service is for. Aspirational role models, when these are unrealistic, can increase social distance, as observed in the phenomenon of beauty magazines that make you feel ugly. The inclusionary quality of role models is in part dependent on the inclusiveness of the role model herself. Simply, health education materials need to represent a realistic image of the people 'like us' who use services, and minimise social distance between the health service materials and the users in order to draw on the inclusionary potential of role models and candidates.

By aligning yourself as distant from a health threat (one that 'doesn't happen to people like me'), an individual can protect their healthy identity, out-group othering the disease and avoiding 'unnecessary' concern. Non-candidacy, or othering the disease, can make health advice personally irrelevant and self-exclude from uncomfortable health guidance (e.g. smoking cessation) and prevention programs (e.g. attending breast screening). Conversely individuals affirming candidacy, particularly where an individual feels fatalism, are more likely to identify and take action on relevant health threats and participate in prevention or detection programs. Fatalism manifests as perceptions of genetic inheritance, or that a disease is 'in the family'; or as a faith-fatalism perception that destinies are in the hands of gods and that human agency is not plausible; indeed to look for cancer was to invite it. If you feel marked, like breast cancer is written on you, because family members have been diagnosed, or because you identify with the 'sorts of women' who develop breast cancer, you are more likely to attend and consistently attend breast screening appointments. In this way, identifying with the health threat and assessing yourself as a potential candidate for breast cancer is an inclusive process, and connects individuals to appropriate health services. Importantly in the case of breast screening, the label (the mark or the disease) is not stigmatised and therefore the othering processes can encourage healthy, inclusive and age-appropriate behaviours. Where the label, or the disease, does have a stigma attached aligning with candidacy may have costs for the healthy identity of the candidate. As commented earlier, the shared cultural knowledge of a stigmatised disease (for example 'avoidable' diseases where the sick become blamed for their own sickness) acts as a cue to the individual, who in turn may resist the disease candidacy and self-exclude from health programs. Disease stigma can also promote secrecy, where the candidate avoids social repercussions of their health threats, by concealing their vulnerability, an example of which is non-compliance with partner contacting schemes in sexual health clinics.

Candidacy does not have to be fearful; awareness of potential candidacy can motivate health protective decision-making and behaviours, such as attending screening, that lead to reassurance and informed management of health risks (Taket and Barter-Godfrey 2005). Identifying with women who can benefit from breast screening becomes inclusionary, increasing attendance and providing the anticipated benefits, either as reassurance or as early detection. Women also identify that noticing changes in their body (not just 'lumps' in the breasts) motivated them to attend breast screening; physical changes remind us that we change as we age, and re-align our candidacy with those requiring breast screening, again including women as service-users who may benefit from the screening service (Taket and Barter-Godfrey 2007).

In this way, those who engage in candidacy, in non-stigmatised and non-fearful ways, and who accept reasonable health threats in perspective of their own vulnerability and capabilities to protect their health, become more included within health services and prevention systems. To an extent, reasonable othering towards yourself that identifies with the need to take precautions can encourage adherence to public health guidelines and promote the inclusion and uptake of services by those who need them most.

Othering, health and inclusive health care practices

By decreasing the social distance between service users and service providers, there can be a greater identification with health advice leading to greater uptake of health benefits of services and behaviours and more inclusive service coverage. However, social distance is moderated by the 'in-group' powerful others and so it is incumbent on the service providers to narrow social distance. Pathways to narrowing the gap include revising practices, campaigns, imagery and representations that are inaccessible to the communities they serve.

Idealised representations need to be balanced against being unattainable or over-aspirational, appealing to the identities of target groups but also offering coherence with their self-perceived capacities for consumption, change and lifestyle choices. In increasingly multi-cultural areas there may be a shift away from photography and literal representations of the target audience to more schematic diagrams as more identifiable and inclusive for a range of ethnicities and cultures. Alternatively, the natural diversity of a community may be reflected in a variety of health promotional materials and services, with tailored messages and programs for under-served groups. In this way, pathways to inclusiveness can be parallel to pathways to equitable health provision. The experiences of health care, as well as how services represent themselves, needs to be culturally competent, to support inclusion and equity. Culturally competent care requires recognition of othering as a power issue for health providers to manage, and respond to by engaging with the othered, connecting with and facilitating reciprocity with out-groups, the stigmatised and under-served communities, challenging othering, stereotypes and stigma, and integrating cultures and diversity of identities in community care (Canales 2000; Canales and Bowers 2001).

At an individual level, competent care needs to recognise similar processes, that people bring complex and sometimes fractured identities particularly in services that see a high proportion of violence and psychological trauma. The value of personal information should not be underestimated; the labelling processes involved in revealing aspects of private lives to health professionals can challenge, reinforce and change self-perceptions and identities. The consequences of revealing or concealing information have ramifications outside the health provision sphere, and professionals need to understand these in able to be able to offer appropriate care. This includes providing ways for people to reveal threatened identities and secrets in a safe and private way that supports transitions of identity and does not marginalise the individual. In particular, health professionals need to respect and value the role that privacy and information control has in the coping strategies of threatened or abused people, whilst encouraging expression of the hurt, abused or violated parts of their life stories. Individually competent care needs to recognise othering, challenge stereotypes and stigma and support the integration and diversity of the clients to provide socially and identity inclusive care.

2.15 Understanding processes of social exclusion: silence, silencing and shame

Ann Taket, Nena Foster and Kay Cook

The greatest triumphs of propaganda have been accomplished, not by doing something, but by refraining from doing. Great is truth, but greater still, from a practical standpoint, is silence about truth. By simply not mentioning certain subjects, ... propagandists have influenced opinion much more effectively than they could have done by the most eloquent denunciations, the most compelling of logical rebuttals.

(Huxley 1946: 12)

Within the context of women's speech silence has many faces ... silence can only be subversive when it frees itself from the male-defined context of absence, lack, and fear as feminine territories ... Silence is so commonly set in opposition with speech. Silence as a will not to say or a will to unsay and as a language of its own has barely been explored.

(Minh-ha 1988: 74)

This chapter considers several forms of silencing. Huxley (1946) explored silencing or the quelling of certain ideas or opinions as an action imposed from above. His exploration of silence and silencing connects strongly to Lukes' second form of power (Lukes 1974), the power to control the agenda. The second form of silencing addressed is that of self-silencing as practised by those whose discipline themselves into being voiceless in order to avoid confrontation, judgement, and as a means of safety (Carpenter and Austin 2007). Last, but not least, this chapter addresses 'unsilence' or the ways in which resistance arises from (and to) silencing. Thus, those who are traditionally silenced gain a voice through subverting and challenging dominant structures and conventions. Feminist author bell hooks (1989) theorises this unsilence as 'talking back'. She represents this notion as an act of defiance, an exercise of empowerment which ultimately shifts the dynamic and power relations between those who oppress and are oppressed, or those who silence and those who are silenced. Examining these forms of silence and silencing is necessary in order to address the creation and recreation of categories which socially exclude and marginalise individuals.

The act or measure of being silenced provides access to limited and/or negative perceptions, causing those who are silenced to be positioned negatively

in normative social and cultural systems. The experience of being marginalised by dominant or normative social and cultural systems is often accompanied by shame. Shame, much like stigma, is often closely connected to
silence and being silenced; as it attaches labels and attributes moral judgement
to the character of those on the margins (Goffman 1963). Those who are
silenced are further inhibited to resist or contest these assignations. When
shame and silencing operate, particular topics, issues or experiences cannot be
voiced, or, are not heard even if voiced (Lorde 1984: 124). The inter-relationship
of shame and silencing is illustrated well in Mizielinska (2001) who examines
the invisibility of homosexual orientation within key texts of the Catholic
Church and the Polish constitution. Consequently, the reinforcing of homophobia and the increasing pressure on lesbians (the particular group in the
study) to remain invisible enacts and imposes shame on these individuals,
allowing their voices to remain unheard in religious and political doctrine.

A counter-position of silence and silencing is the potential to contest and
resist imposed mechanisms of silence, which is seen in 'giving voice' to marginalised groups and perspectives. This counter-silence or 'unsilencing' illustrates how individuals are/become/can potentially be sites of resistance or
contestation, and how silence or silencing can be strategies for re-claiming
one's voice or identity (hooks 1993). Minh-ha (1988) alludes to a subversion
of silence and speech as mechanisms of resistance in her quote at the beginning of the chapter. Thus, silence as resistance is possible. Huby (1997), in a
study of HIV/AIDS care in Scotland, found that her research informants used
silences to serve many purposes, sometimes as strong statements about a person's experience of the services (or the research) as intruding and controlling
and at other times as strategies for coping and survival.

The remainder of this chapter provides examples of interpersonal interactions which construct, organise and perpetuate silence, silencing, shame and
their counter-situations of resistance and contestation. It provides an international examination of these notions with examples from Australia, the UK,
and the USA and emphasises the role of these notions in creating and re-
creating instances of social exclusion. Part 1 of this book drew on social
constructionist and discourse analytic approaches to examine the ways in
which experiences of inclusion and exclusion are mediated linguistically and
culturally in the complex interactions of everyday life, and this chapter draws
on similar theoretical approaches.

These chapter examples are organised along a continuum, beginning with
structural influences on silence, silencing and shame, such as the role played
by the health and welfare systems. Then, we turn to interpersonal interaction
as a mechanism to produce, perpetuate and condone silence, silencing and
shame. For this purpose, we examine intimate partner abuse occurring within
the context of the family. These examples are followed by an examination of
how socially circulated norms and ideals shape the experience of those who
are silenced and shamed. The case of HIV and AIDS discourses will be used
as an example. While we present the above process and products of silence/

silencing and resistance as discrete concepts, the lived experiences of these are messy and interwoven. The following examples provide an exemplar for each type, yet necessarily include reference to the other associated processes.

Shamed into silence: experiences of the LGB community

The first example that this chapter considers is that of silencing as a structurally imposed and mediated condition, although resistible and resisted by those subject to it. The example comes out of a study of the experience of lesbians, gay men and bisexuals in using primary health care services in northeast London (Cant and Taket 2006). The analysis revealed that participants were rendered invisible within the health service, by the assumptions of heterosexuality, as the system, forms and protocols were predicated on heterosexuality. Thus, alternative sexualities were impermissible, thereby constraining the subjectivities of non-heterosexuals. As two different women explained:

> During a smear ... they were asking just really inappropriate questions – 'Are you having sex?' – 'Yes.' – 'Are you worried about getting pregnant?' – 'No.' – 'Why not?' – 'My partner's a woman.' – 'Oh.' [with reported shock].

> My partner went and they asked her about her sex life and about whether she was pregnant and she said: 'No, I'm a lesbian.' and they said: 'Oh, we don't know which of the rest of the questions to ask you'.

Reactions of staff to non-heterosexuality included shock, confusion and an intense refusal in some cases to think outside the box and modify inappropriate protocols, as a third woman in the study reported:

> The GP was adamant, adamant that she was making no referral to a gynaecologist until I'd had a pregnancy test, and I was saying there was no way on earth I am pregnant, and she was saying 'we always do a pregnancy test' ... And anyway she did the pregnancy test and then said, 'you have to ring up for the results', and I didn't, and then I got this shirty nurse who rang me up and said, 'you were supposed to ring up for your results, you're not pregnant', and I said, 'yea, I knew that'.

Throughout the sample it was reported that, except in some specific 'gay-friendly' practices, the environment and procedures of general practices did not acknowledge the possibility that there might be lesbian or gay patients. Some members of the sample reported travelling long distances in order to receive services from health centres and practitioners that acknowledged a wider range of subject positions in respect to sexuality. Lesbians and gay men felt they were being forced to come out when confronted by inappropriate questioning/practices/forms based on an assumption of heterosexuality. They emphasised the unease and discomfort that this caused, particularly at times when they were feeling unwell. It was especially difficult and distressing to first have to break their silence to educate staff regarding the spectrum of human sexuality and its implications for health care practice. They also reported having to prepare themselves for the possibility of shame depending upon the practitioners' response to their situation.

Some women expressed the view that for many of their health problems, it was important that their doctors (and other health professionals) regarded them as women first and when questioning them used language inclusive of lesbianism/bisexuality. One woman talked about the shame she felt when she saw, written across her son's medical notes, 'lesbian mother' implying her sexuality bestowed some terrible pathological risk factor that potentially impacted on or explained her son's health problems. This example highlights the ways in which structures and procedures potentially silence and evoke feelings of shame for members of the lesbian, gay, bisexual and transgender (LGBT) community. It also highlights the risk that breaking silences poses for those in marginalised positions.

Many lesbians/gay men expected the practitioner to ask directly about sexuality and felt encouraged and empowered when this happened. Acknowledgement from the care organisation and practitioners of sexual diversity was seen as directly contributing to the provision of quality, holistic care.

The special clinics and gay friendly practices that do exist create possibilities for open dialogue and inclusion, albeit spatially limited inclusion. The following example, however, provides the converse scenario; one where women experience silencing as an overt and routine policy. Whilst this chapter does not seek to examine structural constructions or experiences of silencing, this example provides insight into the experience of those who are routinely treated as a silenced 'client' of social welfare services.

Silencing from above: single parents seeking welfare benefits

The second example stems from a study of low-income single parents' experiences of the welfare system in Australia (Cook 2005; Cook and Marjoribanks 2005). In this study, 28 women on welfare were interviewed about their experiences of being a welfare recipient. Findings were also compared to an analysis of the *2003–04 Centrelink Information Handbook* (the government agency responsible for welfare provisions).

Centrelink operates from a position where the onus is on Centrelink itself to determine the program and service requirements of the welfare recipient. They state:

> The options approach is a major element of Centrelink's new service delivery model, which has been implemented to provide a high-quality and holistic service to customers. The underlying principle is that when customers come to Centrelink – for the first time or any other time – they will not be expected to know or name the products or services they

may be entitled to. Instead, all they will have to do is truthfully advise Centrelink of their personal circumstances. The onus will be on Centrelink to match the circumstances of the customer with the products and services which have been legislated and made available by Client Departments.

(Centrelink 2003: 2)

The women in this study experienced this approach as silencing. They were excluded from the decision-making process regarding what benefits and services they were entitled to. In effect, recipients were not able to ask for benefits and services that could advantage them, as the case may be that 'they can't ask for what they don't know exists'. As such, recipients were not in a position to suggest alternative programs and services that meet their needs as any part in the decision-making process has been removed. In effect, recipients were subdued and pacified as bystanders to Centrelink's decision-making process. This concurs with statements put forward by Fraser (1989: 174) who contends that welfare recipients are 'rendered passive, positioned as potential recipients of predefined services rather than as agents interpreting their needs and shaping their life conditions.' While Centrelink promotes its role as 'encouraging and enabling people to take part in the community' (Centrelink 2003: 9), an analysis of the roles Centrelink performs, based loosely on Arnstein's (1969) classic ladder of participation, identified their roles primarily as assessing and referring.

Women in the study embodied feelings of silencing, powerlessness and passivity inherent in the Centrelink system:

They [Centrelink workers] do everything to make you feel as powerless and as insignificant and whatever they can. A lot of them are really rude and they've got no compassion or understanding of what you're going through.

They [Centrelink] don't care. They really don't give a shit. I went in there the other day because they were threatening to cut off my pay or I didn't receive a pay and they said, 'Oh, there's something wrong with your form. You might not be eligible for payment.' I went off my nut. I'm like, 'What?' You know. I go, 'so you're pretty much saying that I'm out on the street. I have to live under a bridge with no food, nothing. No clothes, anything on my back and you don't give a shit.' And they're like, 'it's not that we don't care. It's there's nothing we can do about it.'

Very demeaning, very pejorative, they really do. They [Centrelink] need to have respect for people. Yeah, definitely. I know there there's quite a bit of stress with how we go in there and go 'Rah, rah, rah', but it's still. Maybe they're pissed off with the way they're treated. But we're all treated like we're mooching off the dole. Like we're trying to rip off the system. And the more you're treated like that, the more you want to rip off the system.

These examples provide insight into the silenced and shamed lives of women on welfare in Australia. The moral approach (Levitas 1998) to welfare recipients inherent in the Centrelink system demonstrates the power disparity between Centrelink and the low-income women (Cook and Marjoribanks 2005). As Lister notes,

> in any one society the line is drawn in different places for different groups according to the amount of power they can yield. Thus, for example, people with a disability and those in poverty and/or without a home (especially if living on the streets), can find their privacy treated with less respect than that of more powerful groups.
>
> (Lister 1995: 11)

Thus while silencing is practised as a means of rendering recipients passive, there is also the paradoxical practice of demanding great detail regarding the women's lives, for use at the agency's discretion. Again, as with the example of the lesbian mother provided previously, the collection of detailed personal information serves to further silence and pacify recipients who cannot challenge the enormity of data collected about them for purposes they are not privy to.

The next example continues the theme of the experience of service provision, but for a different set of population groups, namely black and minority ethnic groups. Here we examine some examples of a partial service response, offered through the mechanism of special projects/services, outside mainstream health services and often existing on insecure and short term funding, rather than through change in mainstream services. We consider the different practices and patterns of exclusion and the imposed silence it creates.

Partial silencing: ethnic minority communities

Many Somali women refugees have very particular health needs as a result of female genital mutilation (FGM) practices. A focus group was carried out in 2000 with six Somali women who had used the African Women's Advice Clinic in London which was set up to provide advice on women's health issues relating to FGM (Taket 2001). The focus group explored the women's experience of, and views on, the service provided by the African Women's Advice Clinic, as well as their experience of, and views on, their use (or non-use) of mainstream National Health Service (NHS) services in the area.

In particular, the women reported problems that they or other Somali women had experienced in hospital. They reported that hospital staff were not well informed about FGM and responded with shock, surprise, disgust and/or pity. Inappropriate and unhelpful comments, such as 'how did you get pregnant?' were also reported. Such reactions left the women concerned, feeling ashamed and/or blamed for their condition. This should not be taken to mean that practitioners were deliberately rude or offensive, rather that they did not have sufficient information about FGM and know how to respond appropriately to the needs of women who had experienced it. Understandably the women were reluctant to use any services where they feared they would be met with reactions to their circumcisions that would make them feel ashamed or otherwise devalued, and this obviously affects their willingness to use antenatal services in particular. They were thus also excluded from local services, and received further blame and shame for non-attendance at antenatal services. One woman talks about this experience:

> And I think other women, they feel comfortable to talk about that thing [FGM], you know, with X [Somali woman doctor at the clinic], because she already knows, she won't be surprised by what you're talking about. We feel comfortable to go and talk to her if we want, instead of going to the hospital and explain to them and show them you know and they go 'Ooh.' … you feel like embarrassment. When you talk to her, you won't feel embarrassed, you feel comfortable to talk about it. For us we won't go to the hospital to talk about it, for me, I would feel very, very shamed, but with her [X], it is very, very comfortable …

While this example offers a model of good practice for groups with specific needs, this approach responds to diversity by corralling difference into 'special needs' projects/initiatives, thus carrying with it strong messages that reinforce shame, silence and exclusion from 'mainstream' services. Furthermore, projects with temporary or insecure funding help to send the message: your needs are not as important as those of others, marking a different pattern of exclusion.

Taboos, non-existence and silence: intimate partner abuse

The fourth example to be considered addresses the issue of intimate partner abuse (IPA). This example emphasises the function of secrecy in silencing experiences of abuse and the impact of individual silence and silencing in rendering this social phenomenon virtually invisible.

IPA is a major unacknowledged public health problem, with a widespread lack of awareness of the scale and scope of the problem. IPA is not just directed by men against women; partner abuse against men in heterosexual or same sex relationships is also a problem with potential long term health consequences for male survivors (Coker *et al.* 2002), and abuse is also found within lesbian relationships (Tjaden and Thoennes 2000). In a review of 50 population-based studies from 36 countries, it was found that between 10 and 60 per cent of women ever partnered have experienced at least one incident of physical violence from a current or former intimate partner (Heise *et al.* 1999). Research has consistently shown a range of severe physical and mental health problems to be associated with partner abuse (Campbell 2002). Women often say that the psychological abuse and degradation are even more difficult to endure than the physical abuse itself (Heise *et al.* 2002).

Despite the extent and magnitude of the problem, IPA remains a taboo and hidden issue, where individuals are fearful to raise the issue. Women with experience of abuse consult the health service frequently, however health professionals who have not received training about IPA report being anxious or fearful about raising or discussing the issue, citing lack of time, lack of confidence, concern about offending the patient and/or that this was a 'social issue' (Taket *et al.* 2004). Those experiencing IPA are stigmatised and isolated. Their abuse severely compromises their sense of autonomy, self-confidence and self-esteem, and this is reinforced by the societal silence surrounding the issue. Social exclusion is both direct, where movement deprivation is a component in the abuse, and indirect through the lack of open discussion about the issue.

Feder *et al.*'s (2006) meta-analysis of qualitative studies examined how women with histories of IPA want their health care providers to respond to disclosures of abuse. Twenty-nine articles reporting 25 studies (847 participants) were included in the analysis. The women wanted responses from health care professionals that were non-judgemental, nondirective and individually tailored, with an appreciation of the complexity of IPA. Fear that this type of response will not be forthcoming is part of the reason for non-disclosure. Without clear cues from the health care professional that it is safe to disclose, the women remain silent – considering this their safest strategy in the circumstances. Thus in response to the silence of the professional, silence also becomes a strategy for survival. However, in these silences, opportunities for change can be lost: for those who experience IPA to learn they are not alone, not at fault, to receive support from health care professionals and to learn that specialist services exist which can provide information, advice and support.

Women's narratives of their experience illustrate both the hidden issue and their silencing around it, how they often feel unable or unwilling to raise the issue. Some examples taken from Taket *et al.* (2004), a study of the role of English health services in responding to IPA, in which women and health care professionals were interviewed, illustrate the factors at work. One woman narrates a part of her story when she consulted her GP about injuries received from her partner:

> Told him [her GP] I'd fell. ... He didn't quiz me about it. He didn't say anything more about it. I just said I fell and the look he gave was, 'well, I don't think you have, but ... '. I remember sitting there and thinking 'quiz me, quiz me, ask me', and he never did ... because he didn't, I didn't tell.

She makes it quite clear she wants to be asked, directly, and that without this, she is unable to raise the subject. The GP's silence connotes the shame of IPA to the patient, further reinforcing the marginality of her position.

In contrast, a health visitor narrates her experience with a woman who had experienced IPA:

If you ask people – don't pussyfoot around ... I remember when I first plucked up the courage to ask on an antenatal visit. I had never seen this woman before. She wasn't in this particular relationship but she had previously. She gave me the reasons to carry on because she said, 'you must ask everybody. Because I just wanted somebody to come out and ask me.' She lived in a nice house, partner, everything hunky dory, and she were really depressed, and her health visitor kept saying, 'I can't see why you're depressed.' She just wanted someone to ask her. That gave me the reason to carry on asking. I think we need to keep on asking, because they might not tell you the first time you ask them. I don't think I would. So I tell them not to be surprised if I ask them again.

The discussion has focused here on IPA. However, we can find similar dynamics of silencing and exclusion at work in other types of violence and abuse: child abuse, rape and sexual assault, elder abuse, bullying – both workplace and childhood. Providing the opportunity to break silences, as illustrated in this and the next example, can unearth both culturally and socially entrenched silencing as well as provide an opportunity to subvert these accepted norms.

Empowerment out of silence: HIV positive women

The last example illustrates the ways in which silence is countered with defiance, self-reclamation and 'talking back' to situations which enforce or reproduce silence. This example draws on research from the USA and UK, which explored the discourses and representations of HIV and AIDS from health promotion and black women's perspectives (Foster 2007; 2008). Utilising a black, materialist feminist, critical discourse analytic framework, this study examined the discourses and positionalities offered by health promotion information and the discourses utilised by HIV positive black women to represent their experience of living with HIV. The women in this study talked about the silence that surrounded HIV and AIDS, but also, in one of the discourses identified in their talk, the privilege and empowerment afforded by being HIV positive. Women reported 'transcending towards empowerment' as they described taking charge of their life, health and destinies as well as being chosen (often by God) to be HIV positive.

Due to lack of exposure, lack of information or both, HIV is constructed as a disease of 'others', 'deviants' and those external to normal society (Sacks 1996; Singer 1993; Lupton 1994, 1999; Lawless *et al.* 1996; Collins 2000). The ways in which other people perceived HIV and AIDS were discussed at some length by several of the participants. Many of these discussions drew on the deviancy ideology and sourced perceived deviancy to intense and continued stigmatisation of HIV. One woman, Mena, makes a distinction between 'not knowing and discriminating' and 'knowing and understanding' the lives and situations of individuals living with HIV and AIDS. Singer (1993) addresses this construction in her work on the erotisation of HIV as an epidemic of uncontrolled sexual desire which by health and HIV prevention needs to be curbed or restrained. Likewise, Mena connects this sexualisation of HIV and women as prostitutes, contracting HIV through sex with multiple partners.

> They look at you as if you have a bad life; you are a prostitute or something like that. You are a bad person that is it. It has happened to this person, no pity or nothing they just look at you like you are an alien and stuff like that.

Mena also addresses not only how people are perhaps perceived with HIV as being sexually deviant, but also treated as 'others' or 'aliens'. Mena's statement draws on the prevalent representations of women with HIV as sexually deviant, much like the women theorised in Sacks' (1996) and Lawless *et al.*'s (1996) work whereby individual women's lives are silenced and categorised by a preferred stereotype.

In contrast, a construction of HIV as an instrument by which several of the women reported being empowered, enlightened and 'chosen' represents 'HIV as a blessing' illustrating that discourse on religion and spirituality are intricately connected to resisting silence. Below, Gail and Sparky draw on this discourse.

> Researcher: You've mentioned your faith, does that help you cope or deal with being HIV positive?
>
> Gail: Oh, it helps me tremendously because I know that God is in charge. Umm, that umm, that nothing, nothing happens by accident, anything that happens-that happens to me, because he wanted it to, he gave permission for it to happen. Since he permitted it, I just gotta go through it and learn what it is I am supposed to, learn from this experience and help somebody along the way if I can. And I do believe there to be, to be absence and the body to be present with god in the streets of gold. We are all going to die, we know that, and the chances, I probably have a better chance of being hit by a car than dying from AIDS, so, you know. My health, I mean my faith is a big coping mechanism, it helps me get by without having to worry about it. They say if you pray while worry, then why pray. I pray so I ain't gotta worry.
>
> Sparky: Yes, I see people living with it 20 or 30 years, I'm still a newcomer, I just found out in '99 and today, I don't care who know, I'm not ashamed, I'm like hey, this is my testimony, I'm here for a reason, a lot of people have gone on, but evidently there is more work that needs to be done here before I leave and I'd like to be a voice in this world, an example.

Not only do the women's statements reinforce psychological models of coping, the stage or procedural nature of it (Kubler-Ross 1969), but also the higher order appointee or apprentice notion that focuses on divine work and intervention. Their status as an 'example' or 'chosen' has resonance to Biblical discourse which features the trials of martyrs and prophets. They represent this 'chosen' status to afford privilege, as Gail says, she does not have to 'worry' and Sparky represents herself as free and open about her status. Not only does Sparky represent herself as 'an appointee' but also worker for the 'cause,' implying servitude, with privilege associated with divine status. The taking up of such discourse and positionings removes the passive associations of both womanhood and illness. Thus, HIV positive women position themselves as prophets and those with HIV are represented as privileged.

For many women participating in this research study, resisting notions of deviancy for preferred or subversive representations provided an important strategy subverting mechanisms and systems of silence. Resisting these positions of silence enabled them to cope with HIV and AIDS, and potentially aid in the de-stigmatisation of individuals with HIV as well as HIV as a disease.

Conclusion

Looking at a diverse range of groups, this chapter has illustrated the role that silence, silencing and shame play in creating and re-creating patterns of exclusion, fostering localised exclusionary and inclusionary practices and stimulating diverse responses in particular communities of interest.

To finish we want to draw out just some of the implications of these findings for health and human service provision, and in particular for public health and health promotion practice. First of all we note the importance of systems, structures and language – something as seemingly mundane as a health information system or care protocol can reinforce exclusion if it does not adequately respond to the diversity in the populations served. Also important is awareness amongst service professionals of major health issues. Two examples were discussed, IPA, a major issue for all population groups and FGM, a major issue in particular population groups only. Findings here point to the necessity, within the training of professionals, of covering the major health issues as well as the diversity of needs in multicultural populations. Within service providing organisations, a major challenge is that of designing and implementing policies, systems and practices that are inclusive, that respond to diversity rather than creating a limited understanding of majority or 'normal' needs, against which other groups are constructed as deviant with 'abnormal' needs, attracting shame or stigma. It is important to re-orient the mainstream towards inclusivity rather than creating a variety of special case responses that are highly limited in funding and scope.

Part 3

Conclusions and reflections

3.1 Conclusions and reflections

Theory – the seeing of patterns, showing the forest as well as the trees – theory can be a dew that rises from the earth and collects in the rain cloud and returns to earth over and over. But if it doesn't smell of the earth, it isn't good for the earth.

(Rich 1987: 213–14)

Within this book we have *not* set out to provide an all encompassing grand theory that can account for exclusion and connectedness in all their complex and dynamic forms. Rather we have tried to illustrate how exploring the processes that lie behind exclusion and connectedness helps us understand how these arise, and are played out in everyday life. This knowledge helps us understand how practitioners in professions concerned with improving health and wellbeing, and in particular reducing inequities in these, might better shape practice to the achievement of these ends. Our theorising is not produced from some abstract exercise carried out in the academy, as the quote from Adrienne Rich above alludes, it arises from our practice and reflection on that practice, from research into that practice, and we value that mode of production.

We have noted the many different understandings about social exclusion present in the academic literature and within policy discourses. Different definitions of social exclusion exist, each produced in different circumstances, and to some extent, each meeting different needs. Our purpose has not been to craft a detailed genealogy of the term, but rather to illustrate its variety and the necessity of paying close attention to the particular definition(s) that come into play in different policy and practice situations. We have also introduced a number of different theoretical approaches to understanding exclusion and the factors that produce it, and presented the framework that we have found useful in this connection.

The framework we set out in Part 1 has a number of distinctive features in its approach to social exclusion. First, it emphasises social exclusion as: dynamic, multiple and contingent. Individuals, groups and communities usually will experience different degrees of exclusion and connectedness in different spheres of life, and these change through time as external and internal factors change. This complexity demands a nuanced and sophisticated approach to tackling exclusion in both policy and practice. All too often however, responses are situated within the silo of a particular sector, rather than being intersectoral or multisectoral, and are based on a binary distinction between excluded and included. Second, we have emphasised the importance of language in the creation and recreation of exclusion and connectedness. Third, we have emphasised that we find a focus on connectedness (rather than inclusion or participation) as the reverse of exclusion more appropriate in terms of understanding people's experiences. In this short concluding chapter, we consider these features further, exploring some of the implications for policy and practice, drawing on the chapters and research studies presented in Part 2 of the book. We also consider briefly a research agenda for the future.

Responding to dynamics and complexity

We have emphasised the importance of a focus on the privileged, as a distinct group within the broader category of the included. In Chapter 2.1, Pease addressed those of us who benefit most from existing social divisions and inequalities, speaking particularly to white, middle-class, heterosexual, 'able-bodied' men; the chapter illustrated how these inequalities are reproduced by and through the daily practices and life-style pursuits of privileged groups. In Chapter 2.2, Crisp continued this type of analysis in reflecting on her own practice as a social work educator in selecting new students into the social work degree or making determinations about current students. She illustrates how she attempts, through the exercise of professional discretion, to improve social connectedness into spheres of education and ultimately employment for certain groups in the population, such as those with a criminal record. She also identifies how the exercise of such discretion depends crucially on the institutional norms and policies within which she exercises such discretion.

Individual action, interaction and identity are constrained by the operation of institutional norms, practices and policies in ways which can act as exclusionary. Chapters 2.3 by Cook and 2.15 by Taket, Foster and Cook include examples of this in operation in the welfare benefit system and health systems. Chapter 2.10 by Carey *et al.* explores the exclusionary processes applying to voluntarily childless women, illustrating the exclusionary effects of societal norms and discourses about childless women on the experience of those who have elected to be childless.

We have also shown how the experiences of exclusion and connectedness are mediated by different social and cultural factors, whose operation varies across the different levels we have considered: individual, community/local, societal. Some chapters have taken as their focus different communities of interest: carers, considered by Savage and Carvill in Chapter 2.6; immigrants, considered by Renzaho in Chapter 2.9; older people, considered by Nevill in Chapter 2.11; and bisexual young people, considered in Chapter 2.12 by Martin and Pallotta-Chiarolli in relation to mental health and substance abuse. Chapter 2.5 by Owens considers people with disabilities and analyses the issue of access. Although there is a growing awareness of facilitators of access and societal responsibilities associated with these, considerable access issues prevail for people with disabilities. Access is influenced by the processes through which participation is achieved and by the numerous social and structural barriers that compromise participation. A common feature in all of these chapters is the demonstration that the experience of exclusion is a dynamic, rather than a static, phenomenon, and that it can be experienced in a variety of ways – it can be social, financial, educational, employment or service related, or indeed any combination thereof.

Exclusion and connectedness can also operate differently in different spheres of life. Chapter 2.4 by Henderson-Wilson illustrates this with the case of inner city high rise living in Australia, exploring how this particular form of housing can result in both exclusion and connectedness for the residents concerned, and considers the different aspects of the built environment and community activities that can foster connectedness.

Effects of exclusion produced in important areas of health and wellbeing can sometimes be positive and sometimes negative. In Chapter 2.9, Renzaho considers the complexities of the relationship between acculturation and its long-term effect of social exclusion for migrants, producing in some cases deleterious health and social outcomes, whilst in other cases the opposite. In Chapter 2.14, two contrasting examples of 'othering' and marginalisation through being 'the other', were explored. In one case, othering acted as an inclusionary process while in the other it was exclusionary.

Our framework can be viewed as adopting an intersectional approach (Sloop 2005). Intersectionality theory originated in the writings of African-American and third world feminists, concerned to counter Western feminist theory's insufficient attention to women of colour by providing a more appropriately complex and nuanced analysis that incorporated attention to other social-demographic characteristics and the relations of inequality associated with them alongside gender relations (Collins 1991; Mohanty 1991). The main premise that is pertinent here is that any particular form of inequality or oppression is modified by its interactions with other forms or inequality or oppression, and that thus the patterns of exclusion linked to these are similarly modified by interaction. In Chapter 2.1, Pease articulates an intersectional theory of privilege, and shows how this links to the creation and recreation of exclusion. Cant and Taket (2006), in an exploration of lesbian and gay experiences of primary care, showed how a consideration of the intersections of gender, race, class and occupation, together with sexuality was required. They demonstrated how the heterosexist assumptions and systems in relation to sexual health operated with quite different exclusionary effects for lesbians and gay men, and how concerns around mental health resulted in rather different presentations of self for black lesbian and gay men in comparison to those who were white.

A failure to recognise the particularity of the experience of different groups runs the risk of giving rise to what Martin and Pallotta-Chiarolli call 'exclusion by inclusion' where notions of overlap are deployed as signifying inclusion while in reality meaning continued exclusion, through neglect of the non-homogeneous nature of the group and their experiences. An important part of our understanding of social exclusion is that, rather than a dichotomy of included or excluded, there is recognition of long-term processes, grounded in social dynamics and individual experiences that create different patterns of inclusion and exclusion.

Languaging exclusion and connectedness

Throughout the chapters within this book, explicitly or implicitly, the authors recognise that we make sense of the world, our understandings of it, and our place in it, through language; our use of language creates, contests and recreates power, authority and legitimation. Thus language is important in creating and recreating exclusion and connectedness. The specific chapters illustrating this most explicitly are Chapters 2.12 and 2.14.

Building connectedness

Turning now to the question of 'what is to be done' for those who in their professional practice seek to counter exclusion and foster connectedness, a number of working principles can be distilled. The first is the importance of empowerment based approaches; see also Wallerstein (2006), for a review of these specifically in the context of improving health and reducing health inequities. Connected to this is the recognition of the importance of autonomy: 'Autonomy – how much control you have over your life – and the opportunities you have for full social engagement and participation are crucial for health, well-being and longevity' (Marmot 2004: 2). Putting this together with the discussions throughout this chapter on the complex interaction of factors that create and recreate social exclusion, we can note a challenge in terms of building 'real' or authentic involvement for individuals and groups in different arenas of life, in ways that support their autonomy rather than remaining at tokenistic levels. Both these issues are taken up in the recommendations of the report of the Commission on the Social Determinants of Health (CSDH 2008). This will require change on the part of the (relatively) powerful, see Chapters 2.1 and 2.2, and this has been explicitly taken up in some areas of practice, for example anti-oppressive and empowerment practice in social work (Mullaly 2001).

The capacity of information and communication technology to promote inclusion was considered in Chapter 2.7 by Maidment and Macfarlane, who demonstrate how its inclusionary and exclusionary capacities vary across specific contexts at different levels from the most local to the global.

In Chapter 2.8, Stagnitti and Jennings show changes in families' social inclusion which resulted from a program designed to increase the preliterate skills of children by building parents' awareness and confidence, demonstrating some of the careful design that is necessary to craft suitable practice to foster inclusion.

Lamaro, in Chapter 2.13, presents a fascinating example of the implementation of such practice in the challenging circumstances of rural South Africa. The high prevalence of stigma and discrimination towards HIV positive people, and their subsequent experience of social exclusion, has created opportunities for social connectedness through support group participation. This in turn is fashioning an emerging social movement breaking down barriers of stigma, and contributing to broader social change to support HIV action in this diverse and sometimes contradictory social environment.

In Chapter 2.14, Barter-Godfrey and Taket explore 'othering': marginalisation through being 'the other'. The chapter illustrates how othering can operate in multiple ways with both positive and negative effects (and indeed affects), acting as an inclusionary process in some circumstances and an exclusionary one in other circumstances. The implications of this for health care practice were explored.

The organisational challenges that can arise in terms of operationalising these understandings of exclusion in terms of service planning and provision remain to be fully understood. One organisation that has embarked on a systematic exploration of this issue is Wesley Mission Melbourne, a major NGO provider of services in the areas of aged care, counselling, disability, youth, homelessness and employment within the Australian state of Victoria. Wesley Mission Melbourne works alongside those who are most disadvantaged, inspiring them to live their lives to the fullest as valued members of the community. In late 2008, work began with the production of a background paper for the production of an organisational policy on social inclusion (Pollock 2008); this is based on the same framework for understanding exclusion and connectedness that we have discussed, and places emphasis on offering the disadvantaged both voice and choice. Over the coming years the organisation will explore the consequences of this for service evaluation, an initiative to be carried out in partnership with both staff and service consumers.

An agenda for change

Our analysis of how exclusion arises and is perpetuated points to the need for change in both policy and practice. There is a need to move away from 'victim-blaming' approaches that construct exclusion as a deficiency or shortfall in the excluded, rather than arising as a consequence of the complex interactions of a broad range of factors. The growth of critical and anti-oppressive approaches to practice in social work, as well as the growth of empowerment and strengths based approaches in health promotion, public health and other public sector services is a partial response to this, but needs to become more widespread in implementation. This will not be an easy task to achieve, since it demands, in many instances, a change in service ethos at all levels through the minutiae of practice.

As a book written by academics, it would be surprising if there were no calls for further research, and we offer no surprises here. Indeed we do see a research agenda for the future. First in this is a need for more micro-level studies of the dynamic experiences of moving into and out of exclusion and connectedness, to better understand how to foster connectedness and reduce exclusion.

Another element is connected to methodology, in that the types of enquiry that will be particularly informative for re-shaping practice will be those that involve the research participants in wider roles than just the minor role of providing data. Participatory research and participatory action research have a considerable role to play, and the quote that begins this chapter points to our valuing of these research modes. Reflective practice, an organising principle in many of the practitioner fields we have considered in this book, provides a strong basis for research into practice being carried out within practice. The challenge then becomes the dissemination of the knowledge gained beyond the local realm in which it is produced and the integration of knowledge gained from very many small, often qualitative studies. Developments in methods of evidence synthesis (Sheldon 2005; Mays *et al.* 2005), including the application of meta-analysis to qualitative studies (e.g. Noblit and Hare 1988; Schreiber *et al.* 1997; Britten *et al.* 2002; Campbell *et al.* 2003, Feder *et al.* 2006) have a role to play here.

We have discussed the importance of empowerment and strengths-based approaches in practice, and there is a burgeoning literature concerning the development and use of these. Amongst this we find a growing focus on the notion of resilience. A third item in our research agenda for the future is increasing our understanding of the factors that foster resilience, for the individual, family, community or even society. In line with a shift away from victim-blaming, there are dual needs for affirmative research that empowers and celebrates those usually marginalised in research and society, and, for research into resilience and the capabilities and resources that resist exclusion.

The 1990s saw the growth within public health of an explicit focus on human rights as providing the appropriate grounding for public health advocacy into the twenty-first century (Gruskin *et al.* 2007; Blas *et al.* 2008); this has also been taken up elsewhere, for example in social work (Cemlyn 2008). Such grounding is very aligned with the sorts of empowerment and anti-oppressive approaches to practices we identify above. It remains for the future to explore further how such a rights-based approach can assist, and this is an important part of the research agenda we have set ourselves.

References

ABC News Online (2008) 'No doctors found for Tennant Creek', posted Feb. 5 2008 12:32 AEDT. Online. Available HTTP: <http://www.abc.net.au/news/stories/2008/02/05/2154768.htm> (accessed 25 February 2008).

Aber, J.L. and Allen, J.P. (1987) 'Effects of maltreatment on young children's socio-emotional development: an attachment theory perspective', *Developmental Psychology*, 23: 406–14.

Abrams, D. and Christian, J. (2007) 'A relational analysis of social exclusion', in D. Abrams, J. Christian and D. Gordon (eds) *Multidisciplinary Handbook of Social Exclusion Research*, Chichester: John Wiley and Sons Inc.

Abrams, D., Christian, J. and Gordon, D. (eds) (2007) *Multidisciplinary Handbook of Social Exclusion Research*, Chichester: John Wiley and Sons Inc.

Adams, P., Towns, A. and Gavey, N. (1995) 'Dominance and entitlement: the rhetoric men use to discuss their violence towards women', *Discourse and Society*, 6(3): 387–406.

Adams, R.E. (1992) 'Is happiness a home in the suburbs? The influence of urban versus suburban neighborhoods on psychological health', *Journal of Community Psychology*, 20: 353–72.

Aday, L. and Andersen, R. (1981) 'Equity of access to medical care: a conceptual and empirical overview', *Medical Care*, 19(12): 4–27.

Afifi, W.A. and Caughlin, J.P. (2006) 'A close look at revealing secrets and some consequences that follow', *Communications Research*, 33: 467–88.

Agar, M. (1999) 'How to ask for a study in qualitatisch', *Qualitative Health Research*, 9: 684–98.

Ahmad, W.I. and Sheldon, T.A. (1993) ' "Race" and statistics', in M. Hammersley (ed.) *Social Research: Philosophy, Politics and Practice*, London: Sage Publications, pp. 124–9.

Albright, S. and Denq, F. (1996) 'Employer attitudes towards hiring ex-offenders', *Prison Journal*, 76: 118–37.

Alcock, P. (1997) *Understanding Poverty*, 2nd edn, Basingstoke: Macmillan.

Aldridge, S., Halpern, D. and Fitzpatrick, S. (2002) *Social Capital: A Discussion Paper*, Performance and Innovation Unit, London. Online. Available HTTP: <http://www.cabinetoffice.gov.uk/strategy/~/media/assets/www.cabinetoffice.gov.uk/strategy/socialcapital%20pdf.ashx> (accessed 8 October 2008).

Alexander, M. L. (2005) 'Social inclusion, social exclusion and social closure: What can we learn from studying the social capital of social elites?' Paper presented at International Conference on Engaging Communities, Brisbane, Queensland, August 2005.

Alexander, P. and Uys, T. (2002) 'AIDS and sociology: current South African research', *Society in Transition*, 33(3): 295–311.

Alison, J. (2003) 'On receiving an inheritance: confessions of a former marginaholic', *The Way*, 42(1): 22–33.

Allen, R.E. and Oliver, J.M. (1982) 'The effects of child maltreatment on language development', *Child Abuse and Neglect*, 6: 299–305.

Allessandri, S.M. (1991) 'Play and social behaviour in maltreated preschoolers', *Development and Psychopathology*, 3: 191–205.

Alston, M. (2005) 'Drought and social exclusion', in R. Eversole and J. Martin (eds) *Participation and Governance in Regional Development: Global Trends in an Australian Context*, Aldershot: Ashgate.

Alston, M.M. and Kent, J. (2003) 'Educational access for Australia's rural young people: a case of social exclusion', *Australian Journal of Education*, 47(1): 5–17.

Altschuler, A., Somkin, C.P. and Adler, N.E. (2004) 'Local services and amenities, neighbourhood social capital, and health', *Social Science and Medicine*, 59: 1219–29.

Andersen, H.T. and van Kempen, R. (2003) 'New trends in urban policies in Europe: evidence from the Netherlands and Denmark', *Cities*, 20(2): 77–86.

Anderson, C. (2001) 'Claiming disability in the field of geography: access, recognition and integration', *Social and Cultural Geography*, 2(1): 87.

Andrews, M. (1999) 'The seductiveness of agelessness', *Ageing and Society*, 19: 301–18.

Aneshensel, C., Pearlin, L., Mullan, J., Zarit, S. and Whitlach, C. (1995) *Profiles in Caregiving the Unexpected Career*, San Diego: Academic Press.

Anthias, F. (2000) 'The concept of "social division" and theorising social stratification: looking at ethnicity and class', *Sociology*, 35(4): 835–54.

Apparicio, P. and Seguin, A. (2006) 'Measuring the accessibility of services and facilities for residents of public housing in Montreal', *Urban Studies*, 43(1): 187–211.

Archibald, W.P. (1978) 'Using Marx's theory of alienation empirically', *Theory and Society*, 6(1): 119–32.

Arnett, J.J. (2002) 'The psychology of globalization', *American Psychologist*, 57(10): 774–83.

Arnstein, S. (1969) 'A ladder of citizen participation', *Journal of American Institute of Planners* (July), 35(4): 216–24.

Arthurson, K. (2004) 'From stigma to demolition: Australian debates about housing and social exclusion', *Journal of Housing and the Built Environment*, 19: 255–70.

Arthurson, K. and Jacobs, K. (2003) *Social Exclusion and Housing*, Australian Housing and Urban Research Institute, Southern Research Centre. Online. Available HTTP: <http://www.ahuri.edu.au/> (accessed 6 July 2004).

——(2004) 'A critique of the concept of social exclusion and its utility for Australian social housing policy', *Australian Journal of Social Issues*, 39(1): 25–40.

Arthurson, K., Ziersch, A. and Long, V. (2006) 'Community housing: can it assist tenants to develop labour market skills?' *Just Policy*, 39: 13–22.

Atkinson, A.B. (1998) 'Social exclusion, poverty and unemployment', in A.B. Atkinson and J. Hills (eds) *Exclusion, Employment and Opportunity*, CASE paper 4, Centre for the Analysis of Social Exclusion, London School of Economics, 1–20.

Atkinson, A.B., Cantillon, B., Marlier, E. and Nolan, B. (2002) *Social Indicators: The EU and Social Inclusion*, Oxford: Oxford University Press.

Attree, P. (2004) 'Growing up in disadvantage: a systematic review of the qualitative evidence', *Child: Care, Health and Development*, 30: 679–89.

Australian Bureau of Statistics (ABS) (2004) *Australian Social Trends 2004*, Canberra: Australian Government. Online. Available HTTP: <http://www.abs.gov.au/> (accessed 13 February 2006).

——(2007a) *Education and Work, Australia, May 2007*, ABS Catalogue no. 6227.0, Canberra: ABS.

——(2007b) 'More than one in five Australians born overseas', *Media Fact Sheet*. Online. Available HTTP: <http://www.abs.gov.au/AUSSTATS/abs@.nsf/7d12b0f6763c78 caca257061001cc588/ec871bf375f2035dca257306000d5422!OpenDocument> (accessed 25 February 2008).

——(2007c) 'Population distribution, Aboriginal and Torres Strait Islander Australians, 2006'. Online. Available HTTP: <http://www.abs.gov.au/AUSSTATS/abs@. nsf/DetailsPage/4705.02006?OpenDocument> (accessed 25 February 2008).

——(2007d) *2006 Census of Population and Housing* (cat. No. 2914.0.55.002). Canberra: ABS.

——(2008) Feature article 1: Population Projections – A tool for examining population ageing, *1301.0 – Year Book Australia, 2008*. Online. Available HTTP: <http://www. abs.gov.au/ausstats/abs@.nsf/7d12b0f6763c78caca257061001cc588/0046daf21caa349 bca2573d20010fe65!OpenDocument> (accessed 25 March 2008).

Australian Council for Educational Research (ACER) (1997) *National School English Literacy Survey*, Melbourne: ACER.

Australian Institute of Health and Welfare (AIHW) (2006) *Chronic Disease and Associated Risk Factors in Australia*, Canberra: AIHW.

——(2007) *Older Australians at a Glance*, 4th edn, Canberra: AIHW.

Australian Medical Association (AMA) (2002) *Sexual Diversity and Gender Identity Position Statement*. Online. Available HTTP: <http://www.ama.com.au/web.nsf/doc/ WEEN-5HS7D3> (accessed 30 April 2008).

Australian New Zealand Telehealth Committee (2000) 'Telehealth activities overseas', Fact Sheet 4 In *Proceedings of Telehealth Think Tank Melbourne 2001*. Adelaide.

Bailey, A. (1998) 'Privilege: expanding on Marilyn Fry's Oppression', *Journal of Social Philosophy*, 29(3): 104–19.

——(2000) 'Locating traitorous identities: towards a view of privilege-cognizant white character', in U. Narayan and S. Harding (eds) *Decentering the Centre: Philosophy for a Multicultural, Postcolonial and Feminist World*, Bloomington: Indiana University Press.

Baker, K. (2005) 'Assessment in youth justice: professional discretion and use of Asset', *Youth Justice*, 5: 106–22.

Baker, M. and Tippin, D. (2002) '"When flexibility meets rigidity": sole mothers' experiences in the transition from welfare to work', *Journal of Sociology*, 38: 345–60.

Baker Miller, J. (1995) 'Domination and subordination', in P. Rothenberg (ed.) *Race, Class and Gender in the United States: An Integrated Study*, New York: St. Martin's Press.

Ballard, R., Habib, A., Valodia, I. and Zuern, E. (2005) 'Globalization, marginalization and contemporary social movement in South Africa', *African Affairs*, 104 (417): 615–34.

Balsam, K.F. and Mohr, J.J. (2007) 'Adaptation to sexual orientation stigma: a comparison of bisexual and lesbian/gay adults', *Journal of Counseling Psychology*, 54: 306–19.

Baltes, M.M. and Carstensen, L.L. (2003) 'The process of successful aging: selection, optimization, and compensation', in U.M. Staudinger and U. Lindenberge (eds) *Understanding Human Development: Dialogues with Lifespan Psychology*, Boston; London: Kluwer Academic Publishers.

Barakat, H. (1969) 'Alienation: a process of encounter between utopia and reality', *British Journal of Sociology*, 20(1): 1–10.

Barnes, C. and Mercer, G. (2006) *Independent Futures: Creating User-led Disability Services in a Disabling Society*, Bristol: The Policy Press.

Barrett, E., Haycock, M., Hick, D. and Judge, E. (2003) 'Issues in access for disabled people: the case of the Leeds Transport Strategy', *Policy Studies*, 24(4): 227–42.

Barry, M. (1998) 'Social exclusion and social work: an introduction', in M. Barry and C. Hallet (eds) *Social Exclusion and Social Work*, Dorset: Russell House Publishers.

Bartlett, J. (1996) *Will You be a Mother? Women Who Choose To Say No*, London: Virago Press.

Bartolomei, L., Corkery, L., Judd, B. and Thompson, S. (2003) A *Bountiful Harvest: Community Gardens and Neighbourhood Renewal in Waterloo*, Sydney: The University of New South Wales.

Barton, B. (2007) 'Managing the toll of stripping – Boundary setting among exotic dancers', *Journal of Contemporary Ethnography*, 36: 571–96.

Baum, F. and Palmer, C. (2002) '"Opportunity structures": urban landscapes, social capital and health promotion in Australia', *Health Promotion International*, 17(4): 351–61.

Baum, S. (2003) 'Socio-economic advantage and disadvantage across Australia's Metropolitan cities', paper presented at State of Australian Cities National Conference, Paramatta, December 2003.

Bauman, A., Bellew, B., Vita, P., Brown, W., and Owen, N. (2002) *Getting Australia Active: Towards Better Practice for the Promotion of Physical Activity*, Melbourne: National Public Health Partnership.

Becker, H.S. (1993) 'How I learned what a crock was', *Journal of Contemporary Ethnography*, 22: 28–35.

Berman, Y. and Phillips, D. (2000) 'Indicators of social quality and social exclusion at national and community level', *Social Indicators Research*, 50(3): 329–50.

Berry, J.W. (1990a) 'Acculturation and adaptation: health consequences of culture contact among Circumpolar peoples', *Arctic Medical Research*, 49: 142–50.

——(1990b) 'Psychology of acculturation: understanding individuals moving between cultures', in R.W. Brislin (ed.) *Applied Cross-cultural Psychology*, Newbury Park: Sage.

Berry, J.W. and Kim, U. (1988) 'Acculturation and mental health', in P. Dasen, J.W. Berry and N. Sartorius (eds) *Health and Cross-cultural Psychology*, London: Sage.

Bessant, J. (2003) 'The science of risk and the epistemology of human service practice, *Just Policy*, 31 (December): 31–8.

Bessant, J. and Watts, R. (1999) *Sociology Australia*, Sydney: Allen and Unwin.

Beyrer, C., Villar, J.C. Suwanvanichkij, V., Singh, S., Baral, S.D. and Mills, E.J. (2007) 'Neglected diseases, civil conflicts, and the right to health', *The Lancet*, 370: 619–27.

Bhalla, A. and Lapeyre, F. (1997) 'Social exclusion: Towards an analytical and operational framework', *Development and Change*, 38: 413–33.

Bhui, K., Stansfeld, S., Head, J., Haines, M., Hillier, S., Taylor, S., Viner, R. and Booy, R. (2005) 'Cultural identity, acculturation, and mental health among adolescents in east London's multiethnic community', *Journal of Epidemiology and Community Health*, 59: 296–302.

Bigby, C. and Balandin, S. (2005) 'Another minority group: use of aged care day programs and community leisure services by older people with lifelong disability', *Australasian Journal on Aging*, 24(1): 14–18.

Biggs, S. (2004) 'Age, gender, narratives, and masquerades', *Journal of Aging Studies*, 18(1): 45–58.

Biggs, S., Phillipson, C., Money, A.M. and Leach, R. (2006) 'The age-shift: observations on social policy, ageism and the dynamics of the adult lifecourse', *Journal of Social Work Practice*, 20(3): 239–50.

Birdsall, K. and Kelly, K. (2005) *Community Responses to HIV/AIDS in South Africa: Findings from a Multi-Community Survey*, Johannesburg: Centre for AIDS Development, Research and Evaluation.

Blas, E., Gilson, L., Kelly, M.P., Labonté, R., Lapitan, J., Muntaner, C., Östlin, P., Popay, J., Sadana, R., Sen, G., Schrecker, T. and Vaghri, Z. (2008) 'Addressing social determinants of health inequities: what can the state and civil society do?' *Lancet*, 372: 1684–9.

Bond, J., Corner, L. and Graham, R. (2004) 'Social science theory on dementia research: normal ageing, cultural representation and social exclusion', in A. Innes, C. Archibald and C. Murphy (eds) *Dementia and Social Inclusion: Marginalised Groups and Marginalised Areas of Dementia Research, Care and Practice*, London: Jessica Kingsley Publishers.

Bouman, T.K. (2003) 'Intra- and interpersonal consequences of experimentally induced concealment', *Behaviour Research and Therapy*, 41: 959–68.

Bounds, M. (2001) 'Economic restructuring and gentrification in the inner city: a case study of Pyrmont Ultimo', *Australian Planner*, 38(3–4): 128–32.

Bourdieu, P. (1977a) *Outline of a Theory of Practice*, New York: Cambridge University Press.

——(1977b) 'Cultural reproduction and social reproduction', in J. Karabel and A.H. Halsey (eds) *Power and Ideology in Education*, Oxford: Oxford University Press.

——(1985) 'The social space and the genesis of groups', *Theory and Society*, 85(6): 723–44.

——(1986) 'The forms of capital', in J.G. Richardson (ed.) *Handbook of Theory and Research for the Sociology of Education*, New York: Greenwood Press.

——(2001) *Masculine Domination*, Cambridge: Polity Press.

Bowe, F. (1978) *Handicapping America*, New York: Harper and Rowe.

Brehm, J. and Rahn, W. (1997) 'Individual-level evidence for the causes and consequences of social capital', *American Journal of Political Science*, 41: 999–1023.

Brewer, R. (1997) 'Sociology and disciplinary transformation', in J. Belkhir and B. Barnett (eds) *Race, Gender and Class in Sociology: Towards an Inclusive Curriculum*, Washington: The American Sociological Association.

Britten, N., Campbell, R., Pope, C., Donovan, J., Morgan, M. and Pill, R. (2002) 'Using meta ethnography to synthesise qualitative research: a worked example', *Journal of Health Services Research and Policy*, 7: 209–15.

Broady, T., Chan, A. and Caputi, P. (2008) 'Comparison of older and younger adults' attitudes towards and abilities with computers: implications for training and learning', *British Journal of Educational Technology*, 39(7): 1–13.

Brostrand, H. (2006) 'Tilting at windmills: changing attitudes toward people with disabilities', *Journal of Rehabilitation*, 72(1): 4–9.

Brotherhood of St Laurence (n.d.) *Brotherhood of St Laurence History*. Online. Available HTTP: <http://www.bsl.org.au/main.asp?PageId=36&iMainMenuPageId=36> (accessed 29 November 2007).

Brown, R. (2000) 'Social identity theory: past achievements, current problems and future challenges', *European Journal of Social Psychology*, 30: 745–78.

Buchanan, A. (2007) 'Including the socially excluded: the impact of government policy on vulnerable families and children in need', *British Journal of Social Work*, 37: 187–207.

Buck, N. (2001) 'Identifying neighbourhood effects on social exclusion', *Urban Studies*, 38(12): 2251–75.

Burchardt, T., Le Grand, J. and Piachaud, D. (1999) 'Social exclusion in Britain 1991–95', *Social Policy and Administration*, 33: 227–44.

Burton, E. (2000) 'The compact city: just or just compact? A preliminary analysis', *Urban Studies*, 37(2): 969–2007.

Butler, J.P. (1990) *Gender Trouble: Feminism and the Subversion of Identity*, New York: Routledge.

Butler, S., Crudden, A., Sangsing, W. and LeJeune, B. (2002) 'Employment barriers: access to assistive technology and research needs', *Journal of Visual Impairment and Blindness*, 96(9): 664.

Byrne, D. (1999) *Social Exclusion*, Buckingham: Open University Press.

——(2005) *Social Exclusion*, 2nd edn. Maidenhead, Berkshire: Open University Press.

Bytheway, B. (1995) *Ageism*, Buckingham: Open University Press.

Cabaj, R.P. (2005) 'Other populations: gays, lesbians and bisexuals', in J.H. Lowinson, P. Ruiz, R.B. Millman and J.G. Langrod (eds) *Substance Abuse: A Comprehensive Textbook*, Philadelphia: Lippincott Williams and Wilkins.

Caetano, R., Ramisetty-Mikler, S., Vaeth, P. and Harris, T. (2007) 'Acculturation stress, drinking, and intimate partner violence among Hispanic couples in the US', *Journal of Interpersonal Violence*, 22: 1431–47.

Calhoun, C. (1994) 'Social theory and the politics of identity', in C. Calhoun (ed.) *Social Theory and the Politics of Identity*, Oxford: Blackwell.

Callan, V.J. (1986) 'The impact of the first birth: married and single women preferring childlessness, one child, or two children', *Journal of Marriage and the Family*, 48(2): 261–9.

Campbell, C., Nair, Y. and Maimane, S. (2006) 'AIDS stigma, sexual moralities and the policing of women and youth in South Africa', *Feminist Review*, 83: 132–8.

Campbell, C., Nair, Y., Maimane, S. and Nicholson, J. (2007) '"Dying twice": a multi-level model of the roots of AIDS stigma in two South African communities', *Journal of Health Psychology*, 12(3): 403–16.

Campbell, E. (1985) *The Childless Marriage: An Exploratory Study of Couples Who Do Not Want Children*, London: Tavistock.

Campbell, J.C. (2002) 'Health consequences of intimate partner violence', *Lancet*, 359: 1331–6.

Campbell R., Pound P., Pope C., Britten, N., Pill, R., Morgan, M. and Donovan, J. (2003) 'Evaluating meta-ethnography: a synthesis of qualitative research on lay experiences of diabetes and diabetes care', *Social Science and Medicine*, 56: 671–84.

Canales, M.K. (2000) 'Othering: towards an understanding of difference', *Advances in Nursing Science*, 22: 16–31.

Canales, M.K. and Bowers, B.J. (2001) 'Expanding conceptualizations of culturally competent care', *Journal of Advanced Nursing*, 36: 102–11.

Cant, B. and Taket, A.R. (2006) 'Lesbian and gay experiences of primary care in one borough in North London, UK', *Diversity in Health and Social Care*, 3(4): 271–9.

Cappo, D. (2002) 'Social inclusion initiative. Social inclusion, participation and empowerment', Address to Australian Council of Social Services National Congress 28–29 November, 2002, Hobart.

Carney, T. (2007) 'Travelling the work-first road to welfare reform', *Just Policy* 44: 12–22.

Carpenter, L. and Austin, H. (2007) 'Silenced, silence, silent: motherhood in the margins', *Qualitative Inquiry*, 13: 660–74.

Carvill, N. (2008) 'Caring for carers: a theoretical model and assessment tool', Unpublished PhD thesis, Deakin University, Australia.

Cassel, D. (2001) 'Does international human rights law make a difference?', *Chicago Journal of International Law*, 2(1): 121–35.

Cattell, V. (2004) 'Having a laugh and mucking in together: using social capital to explore dynamics between structure and agency in the context of declining and regenerated neighbourhoods', *Sociology*, 38: 945–63.

Cemlyn, S. (2008) 'Human rights and gypsies and travellers: an exploration of the application of a human rights perspective to social work with a minority community in Britain', *British Journal of Social Work*, 38(1): 153–73.

Central Council for Education and Training in Social Work (CCETSW) (1995) *Assuring Quality in the Diploma of Social Work-1: Rules and Requirements for the DipSW*, London: CCETSW.

Centrelink (2003) *Centrelink Information: A Guide to Payments and Services 2003–2004*, Canberra: Department of Community Services.

——(2005) *Centrelink Information: A Guide to Payments and Services 2005–06*. Canberra: Centrelink.

Chappell, C.A. (2004) 'Post-secondary correctional education and recidivism: a meta-analysis of research conducted 1990–99', *Journal of Correctional Education*, 55: 148–69.

Chen, P., Gibson, R. and Geiselhart, K. (2006) *Electronic Democracy? The Impact of New Communications Technologies on Australian Democracy, Democratic Audit of Australia, Report No. 6*, Canberra: The Australian National University.

Cheng, P.S. (2006) 'Reclaiming our traditions, rituals and spaces: spirituality and the Queer Asian Pacific American experience', *Spiritus*, 6(2): 234–40.

Chouniard, V. and Crooks, V. (2005) '"Because they have all the power and I have none": state restructuring of income and employment supports and disabled women's lives in Ontario, Canada', *Disability and Society*, 20(1): 19–32.

Christie, J. (1994) 'Academic play' in J. Hellendoorn, R. Van der Kooij and B. Sutton-Smith (eds) *Play and Intervention*, Albany: SUNY Press.

City of Melbourne (2000) *Housing Survey – New Inner City Residents*. Melbourne: City of Melbourne.

Clark, C. (2005) 'The deprofessionalisation thesis, accountability and professional character', *Social Work and Society*, 3: 182–90.

Clements, P. (2004) 'The rehabilitative role of arts education in prison: accommodation or enlightenment', *International Journal of Art and Design Education*, 23: 169–78.

Coker, A.L., Davis, K.E., Arias, I., Desai, S., Sanderson, M., Brandt, H.M. and Smith, P. (2002) 'Physical and mental health effects of intimate partner violence for men and women', *American Journal of Preventive Medicine*, 23(4): 260–8.

Coles, R. (2005) *Race and Family – A Structural Approach*, London: Sage Publications.

Colette (1966) *Earthly Paradise: An Autobiography*, New York: Farrar, Strauss and Giroux.

Colley, H. and Hodkinson, P. (2001) 'Problems with bridging the gap: the reversal of structure and agency in addressing social exclusion', *Critical Social Policy*, 21(3): 335–59.

Collins, M.F. (2003) *Sport and Social Exclusion*, London: Routledge.

Collins, P.H. (1991) *Black Feminist Thought: Knowledge, Consciousness and the Politics of Empowerment*, London: Unwin Hyman.
——(2000) *Black Feminist Thought*, New York and London: Routledge.
Collins, P.H., Maldonado, L.A. and Takagi, D.Y. (2002) 'Symposium on West and Fenstermaker's "Doing Difference"', in S. Fenstermaker and C. West (eds) *Doing Gender, Doing Difference: Inequality, Power, and Institutional Change*, New York: Routledge.
Commins, P. (2004) 'Poverty and social exclusion in rural areas: characteristics, processes and research issues', *Sociologica Ruralis*, 44(1): 60–75.
CSDH, Commission on the Social Determinants of Health (2008) 'Closing the gap in a generation: health equity through action on the social determinants of health, final report', Geneva: World Health Organisation. Online. Available HTTP: <http://www.who.int/social_determinants/en/> (accessed 10 September 2008).
Commonwealth of Australia (2005) *Budget Paper No. 2: Budget Measures 2005–06*, Canberra: Commonwealth of Australia.
Connell, R. (2000) 'Men, relationships and violence', keynote address to Men and Relationships Forum, Sydney.
Consedine, N.S., Magai, C. and Krivoshekova, Y.S. (2005) 'Sex and age cohort differences in patterns of socioemotional functioning in older adults and their links to physical resilience', *Ageing International*, 30(3): 209–44.
Cook, K. (2005) 'Women, family, work and welfare: a critical analysis of social citizenship', unpublished PhD thesis, The University of Melbourne, Australia.
Cook, K. and Marjoribanks, T. (2005) 'Low-income women's experiences of social citizenship and social exclusion', *Just Policy*, 38: 13–19.
Cook, K. and McCormick, J. (2006) 'Reviewing the concepts of marginalisation and health', in K. Cook and K. Gilbert (eds) *Life on the Margins: Implications for Health Research*, Frenchs Forest: Pearson Education Australia.
Cooley, C.H. (1902) *Human Nature and the Social Order*, New York: Scribner's.
Cooper, R. (2000) 'The impact of child abuse on children's play: a conceptual model', *Occupational Therapy International*, 7: 259–76.
Costello, L. (2005) 'From prisons to penthouses: the changing images of high-rise living in Melbourne', *Housing Studies*, 20(1): 49–62.
Costello, P. (2005) *Budget Speech 2005–06*. Canberra: Commonwealth of Australia.
Cotterell, J.L. (1994) 'Analysing the strength of supportive ties in adolescent social supports', in F. Nestmann and K. Hurrelmann (eds) *Social Networks and Social Support in Childhood and Adolescence*, Berlin: Walter de Gruyter.
Crabb, T. (2003) 'Property: I want a new apartment, baby!', *Australian CPA*, 73(10): 88.
Crawshaw, G. (2002) 'Is there an urgent need for the development of a social model of impairment?', *Australasian Disability Review*, 4: 27–35.
Crewe, M. (2002) 'Reflections on the South African HIV/AIDS epidemic', *Society in Transition*, 33(3): 446–54.
Crisp, B.R. (2000) 'Media advocacy', *Health Promotion Journal of Australia*, 10(2): 105–7.
——(2006) 'Gatekeeping or redressing social exclusion: expectations on social work educators in relation to incarcerated students', *Social Work Review*, 18(4): 4–10.
Crisp, B.R. and Gillingham, P. (2008) 'Some of my students are prisoners: issues and dilemmas for social work educators', *Social Work Education*, 27: 307–17.
Cross, T., Dennis, K., Isaacs, M. and Bazron, B. (1989) *Towards a Culturally Competent System of Care, Volume 1*, Washington: Georgetown University Center for Child and Human Development, CASSP Technical Assistance Center.

Crowfoot, J. and Chesler, M. (2003) 'White men's roles in multicultural coalitions', in M. Kimmel and A. Ferber (eds) *Privilege: A Reader*, Boulder: Westview Press.

Cuhna, M. (2007) 'South African politics, inequalities, and HIV/AIDS: applications for public health education', *Journal of Developing Societies*, 23(1): 207–19.

Cummins, R.A., Huges, J., Tomyn, A., Gibson, A., Woener, J. and Lai, L. (2007) *The Wellbeing of Australians – Carer Health and Wellbeing*, Melbourne: Australian Centre on Quality of Life.

Cyrus, N. and Vogel, D. (2003) 'Work-permit decisions in the German labour administration: an exploration of the implementation process', *Journal of Ethnic and Migration Studies*, 29: 225–55.

Daftary, A., Padayatchi, N. and Padilla, M. (2007) 'HIV testing and disclosure: a qualitative analysis of TB patients in South Africa', *AIDS Care*, 19(4): 572–7.

Daly, A. (2005) *Bridging the Digital Divide: The Role of Community Online Access Centres in Indigenous Communities*, Canberra: Centre for Aboriginal Economic Policy Research, 273/2005.

Davis, C., Leveille, S., Favaro, S. and Logerfo, M. (1998) 'Benefits to volunteers in a community-based health promotion and chronic illness self-management program for the elderly', *Journal of Gerontological Nursing*, 24(10): 16–23.

Day, J.H., Miyamura, K., Grant, A.D., Leeuw, A., Munsamy, J., Baggaley, R. and Churchyard, G.J. (2003) 'Attitudes to HIV voluntary counselling and testing among mineworkers in South Africa: will availability of antiretroviral therapy encourage testing? *AIDS Care*, 15(5): 665–72.

de Beauvoir, S. (1970) *Old Age*, Middlesex: Penguin.

de Haan, A. (1998) 'Social exclusion: an alternative concept for the study of deprivation', *IDS Bulletin*, 29(1): 10–19.

de Souza, P. (2002) 'Flotsam in the migratory wake: relating the plight of the old in Frangipani house and Un Plat de porc aux bananes vertes', *Comparative Literature Studies*, 39(2): 146–61.

de Tocqueville, A. ([1835] 1997) *Mémoire sur le Paupérisme (Memoir on Pauperism)* (S. Drescher, Trans. Vol. 2), Chicago: Ivan R. Dee.

Dean, D.G. (1961) 'Alienation: its meaning and measurement', *American Sociological Review*, 26(5): 753–8.

Dean, H. and Coulter, A. (2006) *Work-Life Balance in a Low-Income Neighbourhood*, London: Centre for Analysis of Social Exclusion.

Department of Human Services (2002) *Neighbourhood Renewal-Growing Victoria Together*, Melbourne: Office of Housing, Victorian Department of Human Services.

De Sandre, P. (1978) 'Critical study of population policies in Europe', in Council of Europe (ed.) *Population Decline in Europe*, New York: St. Martin's Press.

Diamond, L.M. (2008) 'Female bisexuality from adolescence to adulthood: results from a 10-year longitudinal study', *Developmental Psychology*, 44(1): 5–14.

Dickens, C. (1843) *A Christmas Carol*, London: Wordsworth Editions Ltd.

Dillon, P., Wang, R. and Tearle, P. (2007) 'Cultural disconnection in virtual education', *Pedagogy, Culture and Society*, 15(2): 153–74.

Dobinson, D., MacDonnell, J., Hampson, E., Clipsbam, J. and Chow, K. (2005) 'Improving the access and quality of public health services for bisexuals', *Journal of Bisexuality*, 5: 39–77.

Dodge, B. and Sandfort, T.G.M. (2007) 'A review of mental health research on bisexual individuals when compared to homosexual and heterosexual individuals' in

B.A. Firestein (ed.) *Becoming Visible: Counseling Bisexuals across the Lifespan*, New York: Columbia University Press.

Dominelli, L. (2002) *Anti-Oppressive Social Work Theory and Practice*, London: Macmillan.

Donovan, F. and Jackson, A.C. (1991) *Managing Human Service Organisations*, New York: Prentice Hall.

Dreyfus, H.L. and Rabinow, P. (1982) *Michel Foucault, Beyond Structuralism and Hermeneutics*, 2nd edn, Chicago: University of Chicago Press.

Duff, C. (2003) 'The importance of culture and context: rethinking risk and risk management in young drug using populations', *Health, Risk and Society*, 5: 285–99.

Duffy, K. (1995) *Social Exclusion and Human Dignity in Europe*, Strasbourg: Council of Europe.

Dunér, A. and Nordström, M. (2006) 'The discretion and power of street-level bureaucrats: an example from Swedish municipal eldercare', *European Journal of Social Work*, 9: 425–44.

Durant, T.J. and Christian, O. (1990) 'Socio-economic predictors of alienation among the elderly', *International Journal of Aging and Human Development*, 31 (3): 205–17.

Durkheim, E. (1893) *The Division of Labour in Society* (translated), New York: Free Press.

du Toit, A. (2004) '"Social exclusion" discourse and chronic poverty: a South African case study', *Development and Change*, 35(5): 987–1010.

Dyer-Witheford, N. (1999) *Cyber-Marx: Cycles and Circuits of Struggle in High-Technology Capitalism*, Urbana and Chicago: University of Illinois Press.

Easterlow, D., Smith, S.J. and Mallinson, S. (2000) 'Housing for health: the role of owner occupation', *Housing Studies*, 15(13): 367–86.

Edwards, R., Armstrong, P. and Miller, N. (2001) 'Include me out: critical readings of social exclusion, social inclusion and lifelong learning', *International Journal of Lifelong Education*, 20(5): 417–28.

Egeland, B. and Sroufe, A.L. (1981) 'Attachment and early maltreatment', *Child Development*, 52: 44–52.

Eisenberg, M. and Wechsler, H. (2003) 'Substance use behaviours among college students with same-sex and opposite-sex experience: results from a national study', *Addictive Behaviours*, 28: 899–913.

Ellul, J. (n.d.) '76 Reasonable questions to ask about any technology'. Online. Available HTTP: <www.thewords.com/articles/ellul76quest.htm> (accessed 23 January 2008).

Elsinga, M. and Hoekstra, J. (2005) 'Homeownership and housing satisfaction', *Journal of Housing and the Built Environment*, 20: 401–24.

Emslie, C., Hunt, K. and Watt, G. (2001) 'Invisible women? The importance of gender in lay beliefs about heart problems', *Sociology of Health and Illness*, 23: 203–33.

Entrup, L. and Firestein, B.A. (2007) 'Developmental and spiritual issues of young people and bisexuals of the next generation', in B.A. Firestein (ed.) *Becoming Visible: Counseling Bisexuals Across the Lifespan*, New York: Columbia University Press.

Evans, G.W. (2004) 'The environment of childhood poverty', *American Psychologist*, 59(2): 77–92.

Evans, T. and Harris, J. (2004) 'Street-level bureaucracy, social work and the (exaggerated) death of discretion', *British Journal of Social Work*, 34: 871–95.

Eversole, R. and Martin, J. (2005) 'Twin challenges: diversity and exclusion', in R. Eversole and J. Martin (eds) *Participation and Governance in Regional Development: Global Trends in an Australian Context*, Aldershot: Ashgate.

Fabelo, T. (2002) 'The impact of prison education on community reintegration of inmates: the Texas case', *Journal of Correctional Education*, 53: 106–10.

Fairclough, N. (2000) *New Labour: New Language*, London: Routledge.

Fassin. D. and Schneider, H. (2003) 'The politics of AIDS in South Africa: beyond the controversies', *British Medical Journal*, 326: 495–7.

Feder, G.S., Hutson, M., Ramsay, J. and Taket, A.R. (2006) 'Expectations and experiences of women experiencing intimate partner violence when they encounter health care professionals: a meta-analysis of qualitative studies', *Archives of Internal Medicine*, 166: 22–37.

Feldman, L.C. (2006) *Citizens Without Shelter: Homelessness, Democracy, and Political Exclusion*, New York: Cornell University Press.

Fennessy, H., Bound, R., Savage, S. and Bailey, S. (2008) *Parent to Parent 2: A Guide for Parents of Adolescents with a Disability*, Melbourne: Department of Human Services.

Fenstermaker, S. and West, C. (2002a) 'Doing difference', in S. Fenstermaker and C. West (eds) *Doing Gender, Doing Difference: Inequality, Power, and Institutional Change*, New York: Routledge.

——(2002b) 'Symposium on West and Festernmaker's "Doing Difference"; Reply (re) doing difference', in S. Fenstermaker and C. West (eds) *Doing Gender, Doing Difference: Inequality, Power, and Institutional Change*, New York: Routledge.

Ferber, A. (2003) 'Defending the culture of privilege', in M. Kimmel and A. Ferber (eds) *Privilege: A Reader*, Boulder: Westview Press.

Ferree, M., Lorber, J. and Hess, B. (1999) 'Introduction', in M. Ferree, J. Lorber and B. Hess (eds) *Revisioning Gender*, Thousand Oaks, CA: Sage.

Festinger, L. (1954) 'A theory of social comparison processes', *Human Relations*, 7: 117–40.

Filakti, H. and Fox, J. (1995) 'Differences in mortality by housing tenure and by car access from the OPCS longitudinal study', *Population Trends*, 81: 27–30.

Finkelstein, V. (1993) 'Disability: a social challenge or an administrative responsibility?' in J. Swain, V. Finkelstein, S. French and M. Oliver (eds) *Disabling Barriers – Enabling Environments*, London: Sage.

Finlayson, A. (1999) 'The Third Way', *The Political Quarterly*, 70(3): 249–363.

Fish, V. and Scott, C.G. (1999) 'Childhood abuse recollections in a non-clinical population: forgetting and secrecy', *Child Abuse and Neglect*, 23: 791–802.

Flannery, W.P., Reise, S.P. and Yu, J. (2001) 'An empirical comparison of acculturation models', *Personality and Social Psychology Bulletin*, 27: 1035–45.

Fletcher, D.R. (2001) 'Ex-offenders, the labour market and the new public administration', *Public Administration*, 79: 871–91.

Folkman, S. (1997) 'Positive psychological states and coping with severe stress', *Social Science and Medicine*, 45: 1207–21.

Ford, J.A. and Jasinski, J.L. (2006) 'Sexual orientation and substance use among college students', *Addictive Behaviours*, 31: 404–13.

Forrest, R. and Kearns, A. (2001) 'Social cohesion, social capital and the neighbourhood', *Urban Studies*, 38(12): 2125–43.

Foster, N. (2007) 'Reinscribing black women's position within HIV and AIDS discourses', *Feminism and Psychology*, 17(3): 323–9.

——(2008) 'Negotiating HIV health through discourse: an exploration of HIV health promotion and black women's accounts of living with HIV', unpublished PhD thesis, London South Bank University, UK.

Foucault, M. (1976) 'Two lectures', in C. Gordon (ed.) *Power/Knowledge*, 1980, Brighton: Harvester.

——(1978) *The History of Sexuality, Volume 1*, London: Penguin.

——(1980), *Power/Knowledge: Selected Interviews and Other Writings*, C. Gordon (ed.), New York: Pantheon.

——(1982) 'The subject and power', in H.L. Dreyfus and P. Rabinow (eds) *Michel Foucault: Beyond Structuralism and Hermeneutics*, Brighton: Harvester.

Frantz, B., Carey, A. and Bryen, D. (2006) 'Accessibility of Pennsylvania's victim assistance programs', *Journal of Disability Policy Studies*, 16(4): 209–19.

Fraser, N. (1989) *Unruly Practices: Power, Discourses and Gender in Contemporary Social Theory*, Minneapolis: University of Minnesota Press.

Freeman, H. (1993) 'Mental health and high-rise housing', in R. Burridge and D. Ormandy (eds) *Unhealthy Housing-Research, Remedies and Reform*, London: E. and F.N. Spon.

Freud, S. (1930) *Civilisation and its Discontents*, 2002 new edition translation D. McLintock (trans.), London: Penguin.

Gallie, D. (2004) 'Unemployment, poverty, and social isolation: an assessment of the current state of social exclusion theory', in D. Gallie (ed.) *Resisting Marginalization – Unemployment Experience and Social Policy in the European Union*, Oxford: Oxford University Press.

Galvin, R. (2004) 'Can welfare reform make disability disappear?' *Australian Journal of Social Issues*, 39(3): 343–55.

Gammon, M.A. and Isgro, K.L. (2006) 'Troubling the canon: bisexuality and queer theory', *Journal of Homosexuality*, 52: 159–84.

Gardner, I., Brooke, E., Ozanne, E. and Kendig H. (1999) *Improving Health and Social Isolation in the Australian Veteran Community. Research findings from the Improving Social Networks Study*, Department of Veterans' Affairs. Online. Available HTTP: <http://www.dva.gov.au/health/research/isn_study/index.htm> (accessed 1 December, 2007).

Garofalo, R., Wolf, R.C., Kessel, S., Palfrey, S.J. and DuRant, R.H. (1998) 'The association between health risk behaviours and sexual orientation among a school-based sample of adolescents', *Pediatrics*, 101: 895–902.

Garrett, P.M. (2005) 'Social work's "electronic turn": notes on the deployment of information and communication technologies in social work with children and families', *Critical Social Policy*, 25(4): 529–53.

Gaugler, J.E., Kane, R.L., Kane, R.A. and Newcomer, R. (2005) 'Unmet care needs and key outcomes in dementia', *Journal of the American Geriatrics Society*, 53: 253–9.

Geddes, M. (2000) 'Tackling social exclusion in the European Union? The limits to the new orthodoxy of local partnership', *International Journal of Urban and Regional Research*, 24(4): 782–800.

Getup (2007) 'Australia gets up! 07 Post election report', *Getup! Action for Australia* website. Online. Available HTTP: <http://www.getup.org.au/files/Media/GetUpElection Analysis.pdf > (accessed 25 August 2008).

Giddens, A. (1998) *The Third Way*, Cambridge: Polity.

Gillespie, R. (2000) 'When no means no: disbelief, disregard and deviance as discourses of voluntary childlessness', *Women's Studies International Forum*, 23: 223–34.

——(2001) 'Contextualising voluntary childlessness with a postmodern model of reproduction: implications for health and social needs', *Critical Social Policy*, 21: 139–59.

——(2003) 'Childfree and feminine: understanding the gender identity of childless women', *Gender and Society*, 17: 122–36.

Goffman, E. (1963) *Stigma: Notes on the Management of Spoiled Identity*, Middlesex: Penguin Books.

Goicoechea, E.R. (2005) 'Immigrants contesting ethnic exclusion: structures and practices of identity', *International Journal of Urban and Regional Research*, 29(3): 654–69.

Goldberg, C.A. (2001) 'Social citizenship and a reconstructed Tocqueville', *American Sociological Review*, 66: 289–315.

Goldfried, M.R. (2001) 'Integrating gay, lesbian and bisexual issues into mainstream psychology', *American Psychologist*, 56: 977–88.

Goodenow, C., Netherland, J. and Szalacha, L. (2002) 'AIDS-related risk among adolescent males who have sex with males, females or both: evidence from a statewide survey', *American Journal of Public Health*, 92: 203–10.

Goodfellow, R., Lea, M., Gonzalez, F. and Mason, R. (2001) 'Opportunity and equality: intercultural and linguistic issues in global online learning', *Distance Education*, 22(1): 65–84.

Gordon, C. (1980) 'Afterword', in C. Gordon (ed.) *Power/knowledge*, Brighton: Harvester.

Goswami, U. and East, M. (2000) 'Rhyme and analogy in beginning reading: conceptual and methodological issues', *Applied Psycholinguistics*, 21: 63–93.

Gotesky, R. (1965) 'Aloneliness, loneliness, isolation, solitude', in J.M. Edie (ed.) *An Invitation to Phenomenology*, Chicago: Quadrangle.

Gould, L. (2000) 'White male privilege and the construction of crime', in The Criminal Justice Collective of Northern Arizona University (eds) *Investigating Difference: Human and Cultural Relations in Criminal Justice*, Boston: Allyn and Bacon.

Gould, M.I. and Jones, K. (1996) 'Analyzing perceived limiting long-term illness using UK census microdata', *Social Science and Medicine*, 42: 857–69.

Graves, T. (1967) 'Psychological acculturation in a tri-ethnic community', *Southwest Journal of Anthropology*, 23: 337–50.

Grove, N.J. and Zwi, A.B. (2006) 'Our health and theirs: forced migration, othering and public health', *Social Science and Medicine*, 62: 1931–42.

Gruskin, S., Mills, E.J. and Tarantola, D. (2007) 'History, principles, and practice of health and human rights', *The Lancet*, 370: 449–55.

Guillen, M.F. and Suarez, S.L. (2005) 'Explaining the global digital divide: economic, political and sociological drivers of cross-national internet use', *Social Forces*, 84 (2): 681–708.

Habermas, J. (1987) *Knowledge and Human Interests*, Cambridge: Polity.

Hall, E. (2004) 'Social geographies of learning disability: narratives of exclusion and inclusion', *Area*, 36(3): 298–306.

Hall, J.M., Stevens, E. and Meleis, A.I. (1994) 'Marginalisation: a guiding concept for valuing diversity in nursing knowledge development', *Advances in Nursing Science*, 16: 23–41.

Halpern, D. (1995) *Mental Health and the Built Environment: More than Bricks and Mortar*, London: Taylor and Francis.

Halpern, D. (2005) *Social Capital*, London: Polity Press.

Hammel, J. and Finlayson, M. (2003) 'Introduction to the special series on examining the intersections of practice, research, and policy', *Journal of Disability Policy Studies*, 14(2): 66–7.

Han, H-R., Miyong, K., Hochang, B.L., Pistulka, G. and Kim, K.B. (2007) 'Correlates of depression in the Korean American elderly: focusing on personal resources of social support', *Journal of Cross-Cultural Gerontology*, 22: 115–27.

Harding, S. (1995) 'Subjectivity, experience and knowledge: an epistemology form/for rainbow coalition politics', in J. Roof and R. Wiegman (eds) *Who Can Speak? Authority and Critical Identity*, Chicago: University of Illinois Press.

Harding, T. (2005) 'Older people', in C. Harvey (ed.) *Human Rights in the Community: Rights as Agents for Change*, Oxford: Hart Publishing Ltd.

Harness Goodwin, M. (2006) *The Hidden Life of Girls: Games of Stance, Status, and Exclusion*, Malden, MA: Blackwell Publishers.

Harris, B. (2000) 'Seebohm Rowntree and the measurement of poverty, 1899–1951', in J. Bradshaw and R. Sainsbury (eds) *Getting the Measure of Poverty: The Early Legacy of Seebohm Rowntree*, Aldershot: Ashgate.

Harrison, J. and Lee, A. (2006) 'The role of E-health in the changing health care environment', *Nursing Economics*, 24(6): 283–9.

Harrison, M. (1998) 'Theorising exclusion and difference: specificity, structure and minority ethnic housing issues', *Housing Studies*, 13: 793–806.

Hastings, A. (2004) 'Stigma and social housing estates: beyond pathological explanations', *Journal of Housing and the Built Environment*, 19: 233–54.

Hatty, S. (2000) *Masculinities, Violence and Culture*, Thousand Oaks, CA: Sage.

Hatzenbuehler, M.L., Corbin, W.R. and Fromme, K. (2008) 'Trajectories and determinants of alcohol use among LGB young adults and their heterosexual peers: results from a prospective study', *Developmental Psychology*, 44: 81–90.

Havemann, P. (2005) 'Denial, modernity and exclusion: indigenous placelessness in Australia', *Macquarie Law Journal*, 5: 57–80.

Havens, B., Hall, M., Sylvestre, G. and Jivan, T. (2004) 'Social isolation and loneliness: differences between older rural and urban Manitobans', *Canadian Journal on Aging*, 23(2): 129–40.

Hawkins, J.D. (2002) 'Risk and protective factors and their implications for preventative interventions for the health care professional', in M. Schydlower (ed.) *Substance Abuse: A Guide for Health Professionals*, Elk Grove Village, IL: American Academy of Pediatrics.

Hawthorne, G. (2006) 'Measuring social isolation in older adults: development and initial validation of the friendship scale', *Social Indicators Research*, 77: 521–48.

Head, B. (2005) 'Participation or co-governance? Challenges for regional natural resource management', in R. Eversole and J. Martin (eds) *Participation and Governance in Regional Development: Global Trends in an Australian Context*, Aldershot: Ashgate.

Healey, J. (2002) *Self-Esteem*, Rozelle: Spinney Press.

Heaphy, B. and Yip, A.K.T. (2006) 'Policy implications of ageing sexualities', *Social Policy and Society*, 5(4): 443–51.

Heath, M. (2005) 'Pronouncing the silent "B" (in GLBTTIQ)', paper presented at the Health in Difference 5 Conference, Melbourne Australia, 20–22 January 2005.

Heaton, T.B., Jacobson, K.C. and Holland, K. (1999) 'Persistence and chance in decisions to remain childless', *Journal of Marriage and the Family*, 61: 531–9.

Hedelin, B. and Strandmark, M. (2001) 'The meaning of depression from the life-world perspective of elderly women', *Issues in Mental Health Nursing*, 22: 401–20.

Heinemann, A. (2007) 'State-of-the-science on postacute rehabilitation: setting a research agenda and developing an evidence base for practice and policy – an introduction', *Physical Therapy*, 87(11): 1536–41.

Heinrich, S. (2000) *Reducing Recidivism Through Work: Barriers and Opportunities for Employment of Ex-offenders*, Chicago: Great Cities Institute, University of Illinois.

Heise, L., Ellsberg, M. and Gottemoeller, M. (1999) *Ending Violence against Women*, Baltimore: Johns Hopkins University.

——(2002) 'A global overview of gender-based violence', *International Journal of Gynaecology and Obstetrics*, 78 (Suppl 1): S5–14.

Henderson-Wilson, C. (2008) 'Inner city high-rise living: a catalyst for social exclusion and social connectedness?', in *Refereed Papers from the Australian Housing Researchers' Conference 2008 (AHRC08)*, RMIT University of Melbourne, December 2008.

Hershkowitz, I., Lanes, O. and Lamb, M.E. (2007) 'Exploring the disclosure of child sexual abuse with alleged victims and their parents', *Child Abuse and Neglect*, 31: 111–23.

Hertzman, C. (2002) *Leave No Child Behind: Social Exclusion and Child Development*, Toronto, Canada: The Laidlaw Foundation.

Higgins, W. and Ramina, G. (2000) 'Social citizenship', in W. Hudson and J. Kane (eds) *Rethinking Australian Citizenship*, Cambridge: Cambridge University Press.

Hildebrandt, E. and Kelber, S. (2005) 'Perceptions of health and well-being among women in a work-based welfare program', *Public Health Nursing*, 22: 506–14.

Hillier, L. (2007) *"This Group Gave Me a Family": An Evaluation of The Impact of Social Support Groups on the Health and Wellbeing of Same Sex Attracted Young People*, Melbourne: Australian Research Centre in Sex, Health and Society, La Trobe University.

Hills, J., Piachaud, D. and Le-Grand, J. (eds) (2002) *Understanding Social Exclusion*, Oxford: Oxford University Press.

Hird, M.J. and Abshoff, K. (2003) 'Women without children: contradiction in terms?' *Journal of Comparative Family Studies*, 31: 347–66.

Hiscock, R., Macintyre, S., Kearns, A. and Ellaway, A. (2003) 'Residents and residence: factors predicting the health disadvantages of social renters compared to owner-occupiers', *Journal of Social Issues*, 59(3): 527–46.

Hodgson, F.C. and Turner, J. (2003) 'Participation not consumption: the need for new participatory practices to address transport and social exclusion', *Transport Policy*, 10: 265–72.

Holland, J., Reynolds, T. and Weller, S. (2007) 'Transition networks and communities: the significance of social capital in the lives of children and young people', *Journal of Youth Studies*, 10: 97–116.

Holzer, J., Raphael, S. and Stoll, M.A. (2003) *Employer Demand for Ex-offenders: Recent Evidence from Los Angeles*. Online. Available HTTP: <http://www.urban.org/uploadedpdf/410779_exoffenders.pdf> (accessed 27 June 2006).

hooks, b. (1989) *Talking Back: thinking feminist, thinking black*, Boston: South End Press.

——(1993) *Sisters of the Yam: Black Women and Self-Recovery*, Cambridge, MA: South End Press.

Hopkins, L., Thomas, J., Meredyth, D. and Ewing, S. (2004) 'Social capital and community building through an electronic network', *Australian Journal of Social Issues*, 39(4): 369–79.

Horsell, C. (2006) 'Homelessness and social exclusion: a Foucauldian perspective for social workers', *Australian Social Work*, 59(2): 213–25.

Houseknecht, S.K. (1979) 'Childlessness and marital adjustment', *Journal of Marriage and the Family*, 41: 259–65.

Howard, J. and Arcuri, A. (2006) 'Drug use among same-sex attracted young people', in P. Aggleton, A. Ball and P. Mane (eds) *Sex, Drugs and Young People*, London: Routledge.

Hubbard, P. (1998) 'Community action and the displacement of street prostitution: evidence from British cities', *Geoforum*, 29: 269–86.

Huby, G. (1997) 'Interpreting silence, documenting experience: an anthropological approach to the study of health service users' experience with HIV/AIDS care in Lothian, Scotland', *Social Science and Medicine*, 44: 1149–60.

Huddy, L. (2007) 'From social to political identity: a critical examination of Social Identity Theory', *Political Psychology*, 22: 127–56.

Huebner, C.E. (2000) 'Community-based support for preschool readiness among children in poverty', *Journal of Education for Students Placed at Risk*, 5: 291–314.

Hughes, T.L. and Eliason, M. (2002) 'Substance use and abuse in lesbian, gay bisexual and transgender populations', *Journal of Primary Prevention*, 22: 263–98.

Hull, A. (2006) 'Facilitating structures for neighbourhood regeneration in the UK: the contribution of the Housing Action Trusts', *Urban Studies*, 43(12): 2317–50.

Humpage, L. (2006) 'An "inclusive" society: a "leap forward" for Maori in New Zealand?' *Critical Social Policy*, 26(1): 220–42.

Hunt, L.M., Schneider, S. and Comer, B. (2004) 'Should "acculturation" be a variable in health research? A critical review of research on US Hispanics', *Social Science and Medicine*, 59: 973–86.

Hunter, S., Wong, M., Beighley, C. and Morral, A. (2006) 'Acculturation and driving under the influence: a study of repeat offenders', *Journal of Studies on Alcohol*, 67: 458–64.

Hurst, C. (2001) *Social Inequality: Forms, Causes and Consequences*, 4th edn, Boston: Allyn and Bacon.

Hutchinson, P. and Mahlalela, X. (2006) 'Utilization of voluntary counselling and testing services in the Easter Cape, South Africa', *AIDS Care*, 18(5): 446–55.

Hutchison, T. (2007) 'Listen up, Senator, we won't forgive', *The Age*, Melbourne, 5 May 2007: 9.

Huxley, A. (1946) *Brave New World*, Harmondsworth: Penguin.

Iliffe, J. (2006) *The African AIDS Epidemic: A History*, Oxford: James Currey.

Imrie, R. (2003) 'Housing quality and the provision of accessible homes', *Housing Studies*, 18(3): 387–408.

Internet World Stats (2007) Usage and Population Statistics. Online. Available HTTP: <http://www.internetworldstats.com/stats6.htm> (accessed 9 July 2007).

Ireland, M. (1993) *Reconceiving Women: Separating Motherhood from Female Identity*, New York: Guilford.

Jaber, L., Brown, M., Hammad, A., Zhu, Q. and Herman, W.H. (2003) 'Lack of acculturation is a risk factor for diabetes in Arab immigrants in the US', *Diabetes Care*, 26: 2010–14.

Jalving, C. (n.d.) *Nostalgia, Reverie and Intoxicating Dreams. Romantic Longing in the Art of Peter Callesen*. Online. Available HTTP: http://www.petercallesen.com/index/texts.htm (accessed 25 March 2008).

Jamrozik, A. and Nocella, L. (1998) *The Sociology of Social Problems: Theoretical Perspectives and Methods of Intervention*, Melbourne: Cambridge University Press.

Jarman, J. (2001) 'Explaining social exclusion', *International Journal of Sociology and Social Policy*, 21(4): 3–9.

Jennings, C. and Stagnitti, K. (2007) 'From little things big things grow', *EQ Australia*, Autumn: 34–6.

Jensen, J.L. (2003) 'Virtual democratic dialogue? Bringing together citizens and politicians', *Information Polity*, 8, 29–47.

Jewkes, R. (2006) 'Beyond stigma: social responses to HIV in South Africa', *The Lancet*, 368: 430–1.

Johnson, A. (2001) *Privilege, Power and Difference*, Mountain View, CA: Mayfield Publishing Company.

Johnson, J., Farrell, W. and Stoloff, J. (2000) 'An empirical assessment of four perspectives on the declining fortunes of the African-American male', *Urban Affairs Review*, 35: 695–716.

Johnson, J.L., Bottorff, J.L., Browne, A.J., Grewal, S., Hilton, B.A. and Clarke, H. (2004) 'Othering and being othered in the context of health care services', *Health Communication*, 16: 253–71.

Johnson, M.A., Chow, J.C-C., Ketch, V. and Austin, M.J. (2006) 'Implementing welfare-to-work decisions: a study of staff decision-making', *Families in Society*, 87: 317–25.

Jones, A. and Smythe, P. (1999) 'Social exclusion: a new framework for social policy analysis', *Just Policy*, 17: 11–20.

Jordan, B. (2001) 'Tough love: social work, social exclusion and the third way', *British Journal of Social Work*, 31(4): 527–46.

Jones, P.S. (2005) '"A test of governance": rights-based struggles and the politics of HIV/AIDS policy in South Africa', *Political Geography*, 24: 419–47.

Jones, T., Savage, S., Bailey, S., Bound, R., Boyd, G. and Lavery, J. (2003) *Parent to Parent. Raising your Child with Special Needs*, Geelong: Deakin University and Department of Human Services (Barwon-South Western Region).

Jorm, A.F, Korten, A.E., Rodgers, B., Jacomb, P.A. and Christensen, H. (2002) 'Sexual orientation and mental health: results from a community survey of young and middle-aged adults', *British Journal of Psychiatry*, 180: 423–7.

Josephs, R.A., Markus, H.R. and Tafarodi, R.W. (1992) 'Gender and self-esteem', *Journal of Personality and Social Psychology*, 63: 391–402.

Judd, B. and Randolph, B. (2006) 'Qualitative methods and the evaluation of community renewal programs in Australia: towards a national framework', *Urban Policy and Research*, 24(1): 97–114.

Judd, B., Samuels, R. and O'Brien, E. (2002) *Linkages Between Housing Policing and Other Interventions for Crime and Harassment Reduction on Public Housing Estates*. Positioning Paper, Melbourne: Australian Housing and Urban Research Institute. Online. Available HTTP: <www.ahuri.com/> (accessed 4 October 2003).

Judge, J. and Bauld, L. (2006) 'Learning from failure? Health Action Zones in England', *European Journal of Public Health*, 16(4): 341–4.

Jung, C.G. (1961) *Memories, Dreams, Reflections*, 1995 reprint, London: Fontana.

Kabeer, N. (2006) 'Social exclusion and the MDGs: the challenge of "durable inequalities" in the Asian context', in Asia 2015 – Promoting Growth Ending Poverty, Institute of Development Studies. Online. Available HTTP: <http://www.asia2015 conference.org/pdfs/Kabeer.pdf> (accessed 2 August 2007).

Kamineni, A., Williams, M., Schwartz, S., Cook, L. and Weiss, N. (1999) 'The incidence of gastric carcinoma in Asian migrants to the United States and their descendants', *Cancer Causes Control*, 10: 77–83.

Karlsson, H. (2007) 'Stigma and humiliation – unfortunately close friends' *Nordic Journal of Psychiatry*, 61: 5.

Kauffman, K. and Lindauer, D. (2004) *AIDS and South Africa: the Social Expression of a Pandemic*, New York: Palgrave Macmillan.

Kawachi, I. and Berkman, L. (2000) 'Chapter 8: social cohesion, social capital, and health', in L.F. Berkman and I. Kawachi (eds) *Social Epidemiology*, Oxford: Oxford University Press.

Keizer, R., Dykstra, P.A. and Jansen, M.D. (2007) 'Pathways into childlessness: evidence of gendered life discourse dynamics', *Journal of Biosocial Science*, 39: 1–16.

Kelly, K.J. and Van Vlaenderen, H. (1996) 'Dynamics of participation in a community health project', *Social Science and Medicine*, 42(9): 1235–46.

Kenna, T.E. (2007) 'Consciously constructing exclusivity in the suburbs? Unpacking a master planned estate development in western Sydney', *Geographical Research*, 45 (3): 300–13.

Keniston, K. (1972) 'The varieties of alienation: an attempt at definition', in A.W. Finifter (ed.) *Alienation and the Social System*, New York: John Wiley and Sons, Inc.

Kessler, E-M. and Staudinger, U.M. (2007) 'Intergenerational potential: effects of social interaction between older adults and adolescents', *Psychology and Aging*, 22 (4): 690–704.

Khakee, A., Somma, P. and Thomas, H. (eds) (1999) *Urban Renewal, Ethnicity and Social Exclusion in Europe*, Aldershot: Ashgate.

Kilcannon, C.L., He, W. and West, L.A. (2005) 'Demography of aging in China and the United States and the economic well-being of their older populations', *Journal of Cross-Cultural Gerontology*, 20: 243–55.

Kim, I.K. and Kim, C-S. (2003) 'Patterns of family support and the quality of life of the elderly', *Social Indicators Research*, 62(1): 437–54.

Kim, J. and Kaplan, R. (2004) 'Physical and psychological factors in sense of community: new urbanist Kentlands and nearby Orchard Village', *Environment and Behavior*, 36(3): 313–40.

King, M. and McKeown, E. (2003) *Mental Health and Social Wellbeing of Gay Men, Lesbians and Bisexuals in England and Wales*, London: Mind (National Association for Mental Health).

Kitchin, R. (1998) '"Out of place", "Knowing one's place": space, power and the exclusion of disabled people', *Disability and Society*, 13(3): 343–56.

Kitchin, R. and Law, R. (2001) 'The socio-spatial construction of (in)accessible public toilets', *Urban Studies*, 38(2): 287–98.

Kitchin, R. and Lysaght, K. (2004) 'Sexual citizenship in Belfast, Northern Ireland', *Gender, Policy and Culture*, 11(1): 84–103.

Kitchin, R., Shirlow, P. and Shuttleworth, I. (1998) 'On the margins: disabled people's experience of employment in Donegal, West Ireland', *Disability and Society*, 13(5): 785–806.

Klasen, S. (n.d.) *Social exclusion, Children, and Education: Conceptual and Measurement Issues, Department of Economics*, University of Munich. Online. Available HTTP: <http://www.oecd.org/dataoecd/19/37/1855901.pdf> (accessed 10 October 2008).

Knipscheer, J. and Kleber, R. (2007) 'Acculturation and mental health among Ghanaians in the Netherlands', *International Journal of Social Psychiatry*, 53: 369–83.

Kobayashi, K.M. (2000) 'The nature of support from adult *sansei* (third generation) children to older *nisei* (second generation) parents in Japanese Canadian families', *Journal of Cross-Cultural Gerontology*, 15: 185–205.

Koch, P. (1994) *Solitude: A Philosophical Encounter*, La Salle, Illinois: Open Court.

Kubler-Ross, E. (1969) *On Death and Dying*, New York: Macmillan.

Kutza, E.A. (2005) 'The intersection of economics and family status in late life: implications for the future', *Marriage and Family Review*, 37(1/2): 9.

Kweon, B., Sullivan, W.C. and Wiley, A.R. (1998) 'Green common spaces and the social integration of inner-city older adults', *Environment and Behavior*, 30(6): 832–59.

Labonte, R. (2004) 'Social inclusion/exclusion: dancing the dialectic', *Health Promotion International*, 19(1): 115–21.

Lawless, S., Kippax, S. and Crawford, J. (1996) 'Dirty, diseased and undeserving: the positioning of HIV positive women', *Social Science and Medicine*, 43: 1371–7.

Lawrence, R.J. (2005) 'Chapter 1: Methodologies in contemporary housing research: a critical review', in D.U. Vestbro, Y. Hurol and N. Wilkinson (eds) *Methodologies in Housing Research*, Great Britain: The Urban International Press.

Lee, R., Kochman, K. and Sikkema, K. (2002) 'Internalised stigma among people living with HIV-AIDS', *AIDS and Behaviour*, 6(4): 309–19.

Lee, Y. and Mittelstaedt, R. (2004) 'Impact of injury level and self-monitoring on free time boredom of people with spinal cord injury', *Disability and Rehabilitation*, 26 (19): 1143–9.

Lenoir, R. (1974/1989) *Les Exclus: Un Francais sur Dix*, 2nd ed. Paris: Editions du Seuil.

Leonard, M. (2004) 'Bonding and bridging capital: reflections from Belfast', *Sociology*, 38(5): 927–44.

Leong, F.T. and Chou, E.L. (1994) 'The role of ethnic identity and acculturation in the vocational behaviour of Asian Americans. An integrative review', *Journal of Vocational Behavior*, 44: 155–72.

Letherby, G. (1994) 'Mother or not, mother or what? Problems of definition and identity', *Women's Studies International Forum*, 17: 525–32.

——(1999) 'Other than mother and mothers as others: the experience of motherhood and non-motherhood in relation to "infertility" and "involuntary childlessness"', *Women's Studies International Forum*, 22: 359–72.

——(2000) 'Images and representations of non-motherhood', *Reproductive Health Matters*, 8: 143.

——(2002) 'Childless and bereft? Stereotypes and realities in relation to "voluntary" and "involuntary" childlessness and womanhood', *Sociological Inquiry*, 72: 7–20.

Letherby, G. and Williams, C. (1999) 'Non-motherhood: ambivalent autobiographies', *Feminist Studies*, 25: 719–28.

Levitas, R. (1998) *The Inclusive Society? Social Exclusion and New Labour*, London: Macmillan.

——(2004) 'Let's hear it for Humpty': social exclusion, the third way and cultural capital, *Cultural Trends*, 13(2): 41–56.

——(2005) *The Inclusive Society? Social Exclusion and New Labour*, 2nd edn, London: Palgrave Macmillan.

Levitas, R., Pantazis, C., Fahmy, E., Gordon, D., Lloyd, E. and Patsios, D. (2007) *The Multi-Dimensional Analysis of Social Exclusion*, Bristol: Department of Sociology and School for Social Policy, University of Bristol.

Leyden, K.M. (2003) 'Social capital and the built environment: the importance of walkable neighbourhoods', *American Journal of Public Health*, 9(9): 1546–51.

Lin, N. (2001) *Social Capital: A Theory of Social Structure and Action*, New York: Cambridge University Press.

Link, B.G. and Phelan, J.C. (2001a) *On Stigma and its Public Health Implications*. Maryland: National Institutes of Health. Online. Available HTTP: <http://www.stigmaconference.nih.gov/FinalLinkPaper.html> (accessed 29 July 2006).

——(2001b) 'Conceptualizing stigma', *Annual Review of Sociology*, 27: 363–85.

——(2006) 'Stigma and its public health implications', *Lancet*, 376: 528–9.

Link, B.G., Yang, L.H., Phelan, J.C. and Collins, P.Y. (2004) 'Measuring mental illness stigma', *Schizophrenia Bulletin*, 30: 511–41.

Lipsky, R. (1980) *Street Level Bureaucracy: Dilemmas of the Individual in Public Services*, New York: Russell Sage Foundation.

Lister, R. (1995) 'Dilemmas in engendering citizenship', *Economy and Society*, 24(1): 1–40.

——(1997) *Citizenship: Feminist Perspectives*, Houndsmills: Macmillan.

——(2000) 'Strategies for social inclusion: promoting social cohesion or social justice', in P. Askonas and A. Stewart (eds) *Social Inclusion: Possibilities and Tensions*, London: Macmillan.

Litt, J., Gaddis, B.J., Needles Fletcher, C. and Winter, M. (2000) 'Leaving welfare: independence or continued vulnerability?' *The Journal of Consumer Affairs*, 34: 82–96.

Llewellyn, P. (2007) 'Reporting research: using the views of people with learning disabilities', *Learning Disability Practice*, 10(1): 28–31.

Lloyd, R. and Hellwig, O. (2000) *Barriers to the Uptake of New Technology, Discussion Paper No.53*. Canberra: NATSEM.

López, E.J., Ehly, S. and García-Vásquez, E. (2002) 'Acculturation, social support and academic achievement of Mexican and Mexican American high school students: an exploratory study', *Psychology in the Schools*, 39: 245–257.

Lorde, A. (1984) *Sister Outsider*, Trumansburg, NY: Crossing Press.

Loughlin, D., Simon-Rusinowitz, L., Mahoney, K., Desmond, S., Squillace, M. and Powers, L. (2004) 'Preferences for a cash option versus traditional services for Florida children and adolescents with developmental disabilities', *Journal of Disability Policy Studies*, 14(4): 229–40.

Lukes, S. (1974) *Power: A Radical View*, London: Macmillan.

——(1997) 'Toleration and recognition', *Ratio Juris*, 10(2): 213–22.

Lupton, D. (1994) *Moral Threats and Dangerous Desires: AIDS in the News Media*, London: Taylor Francis.

Lupton, D. (1999) 'Archetypes of infection: people with HIV/AIDS in the Australian press in the mid 1990s', *Sociology of Health and Illness*, 21(1): 37–53.

Lutz, M.A. (2002) 'Social economics, justice and the common good', *International Journal of Social Economics*, 29 (1/2): 26–44.

Lyn, K. (1992) 'White privilege: what's in it for me?' in C. James and A. Shadd (eds) *Talking About Difference: Encounters in Culture, Language and Identity*, Toronto: Between the Lines Press.

Lyon, T.D. (1996) 'The effects of threats on children's disclosure of sexual abuse', *The APSAC Advisor*, 9: 9–15.

McAllister, F. and Clark, L. (1998) *Choosing Childlessness: Family and Parenthood, Policy and Practice*, London: Routledge.

McCabe, S.E., Boyd, C., Hughes, T.L. and d'Arcy, H. (2003) 'Sexual identity and substance abuse among undergraduate students', *Substance Abuse*, 24(2): 77–91.

McCain, M. and Mustard, J.F. (1999) *Reversing the Real Brain Drain: Early Years Study Final Report*, Toronto: The Founders' Network of the Canadian Institute for Advanced Research.

——(2002) *The Early Years Study: Three Years Later*, Toronto: The Founders' Network of the Canadian Institute for Advanced Research.

McCarty, D. and Clancy, C. (2002) 'Telehealth: implications for social work practice', *Social Work*, 47(2): 153–61.

MacDonald, R. (ed.) (2004) *Youth, the Underclass and Social Exclusion*, London: Routledge.

McDonald, C., Marston, G. and Buckley, A. (2003) 'Risk technology in Australia: the role of the job seeker classification instrument in employment services', *Critical Social Policy*, 23(4): 498–525.

McDougall, J., DeWit, D., King, G., Mille, L. and Killip, S. (2004) 'High school-aged youths attitudes toward their peers with disabilities: the role of school and student interpersonal factors', *International Journal of Disability, Development and Education*, 51(3): 287–313.

McDowell, L. (2000) 'The trouble with men? Young people, gender transformations and the crisis of masculinity', *International Journal of Urban and Regional Research*, 24(1): 201–9.

McDowell, L., Ward, K., Perrons, D., Ray, K. and Fagan, C. (2006) 'Place, class and local circuits of reproduction: exploring the social geography of middle-class childcare in London', *Urban Studies*, 43(12): 2163–82.

Macintyre, S., Ellaway, A., Hiscock, R., Kearns, A., Der, G. and McKay, L. (2003) 'What features of the home and the area might help to explain observed relationships between housing tenure and health? Evidence from the west of Scotland', *Health and Place*, 9: 207–18.

McKenzie, K. (2007) 'Digital divides: the implications for social inclusion', *Learning Disability Practice*, 10(6): 16–21.

MacLachlan, M. (1997) *Culture and Health*, Chichester: John Wiley and Sons Ltd.

McLean, K. (2001) 'Living life in the double closet: young bisexuals speak out', *Hecate*, 27(1): 109–18.

——(2008) 'Inside, outside, nowhere: bisexual men and women in the gay and lesbian community', *Journal of Bisexuality*, 8(1–2): 63–80.

McLoyd, V.C. (1998) 'Socioeconomic disadvantage and child development', *American Psychologist*, 53: 185–204.

McMillen, A. and Soderberg, S. (2002) 'Disabled persons' experience of dependence on assistive devices', *Scandinavian Journal of Occupational Therapy*, 9(4): 176–83.

McNelis, S. and Reynolds, A. (2001) *Creating Better Futures for Residents of Highrise Public Housing in Melbourne*, Melbourne: Ecumenical Housing Inc.

McNutt, J.G. and Menon, G.M. (2008) 'The rise of cyberactivism: implications for the future of advocacy in the human services', *Families in Society*, 89(1): 33–8.

McQuaid, R.W., Lindsay, C. and Greig, M. (2004) '"Reconnecting" the unemployed: information and communication technology and services for jobseekers in rural areas', *Information, Communication and Society*, 7(3): 364–88.

Magen, R.H. and Emerman, J. (2000) 'Should convicted felons be denied admission to a social work education program? Yes!' *Journal of Social Work Education*, 36: 401–5.

Magliano, L., Fadden, G., Madianos, M., de Almeida, J., Held, T., Guarneri, M., Narascim C., Tosini, P. and Maj, M. (1998) 'Burden on the families of patients with schizophrenia: results of the BIOMED I study', *Social Psychiatry and Psychiatric Epidemiology*, 33: 405–12.

Mainous, A., Majeed, A., Koopman, R., Baker, R., Everett, C., Tilley, B. and Diaz, V. (2006) 'Acculturation and diabetes among Hispanics: evidence from the 1999–2002 National Health and Nutrition Examination Survey', *Public Health Reports*, 121: 60–6.

Mair, G. and May, C. (1997) *Offenders on Probation*, London: Home Office.

Makin, L. and Diaz, C.J. (2004) *Literacies in Early Childhood: Changing Views Challenging Practice*, Sydney: MacLennan and Petty.

Maldonado, L. (2002) 'Symposium on West and Fenstermaker's "Doing Difference"', in S. Fenstermaker and C. West (eds) *Doing Difference, Doing Gender: Inequality, Power and Institutional Change*, New York: Routledge.

Marino, R., Stuart, S., Wright, C., Minas, H. and Klimidis, S. (2001) 'Acculturation and dental health among Vietnamese living in Melbourne, Australia', *Community Dentistry and Oral Epidemiology*, 29: 107–110.

Markham, A.N. (2005) 'The methods, politics, and ethics of representation in online ethnography', in N. Denzin and Y. Lincoln (eds) *The Sage Handbook of Qualitative Research*, Thousand Oaks, CA: Sage.

Marks, G., Solis, J., Richardson, J.L., Collins, L.M., Birba, L. and Hisserich, J.C. (1987) 'Health behavior of elderly Hispanic women: does cultural assimilation make a difference?' *American Journal of Public Health*, 77: 1315–19.

Marmot, M. (2004) *Status Syndrome: How Your Social Standing Directly Affects your Health*, London: Bloomsbury.

Marsh, A. and Mullins, D. (1998) 'The social exclusion perspective and housing studies: origins, applications and limitations', *Housing Studies*, 13(4): 749–60.

Marshall, T.H. (1950) *Citizenship and Social Class*, Cambridge: Cambridge University Press.

Martens, A., Goldenberg, J.L. and Greenberg, J. (2005) 'A Terror Management Perspective on Ageism', *Journal of Social Issues*, 61(2): 223–39.

Martin, E. (2007) 'Exploring mental health in relation to substance use and abuse amongst bisexual youth', Unpublished Bachelor of Applied Science (Health Promotion) Honours thesis, Deakin University, Australia.

Martin, S. (2004) 'Reconceptualising social exclusion: a critical response to the neo-liberal welfare reform agenda and the underclass thesis', *Australian Journal of Social Issues*, 39: 79–94.

Marx, K. (1894; 1999) *Capital: An Abridged Edition*, Oxford: Oxford World's Classics, Oxford University Press.

Mays, N., Pope, C. and Popay, J. (2005) 'Systematically reviewing qualitative and quantitative evidence to inform management and policy-making in the health field', *Journal of Health Services Research and Policy*, 10 (Suppl 1): S1:6–20.

Meeks, C.B., Nickols, S.Y. and Sweaney, A.L. (1999) 'Demographic comparisons of aging in five selected countries', *Journal of Family and Economic Issues*, 20(3): 223–50.

Meikle, G. (2004) 'Networks of influence: internet activism in Australia and beyond', in G. Goggin (ed.) *Virtual Nation: The Internet in Australia*, Sydney: UNSW Press.

Mendes, P. (2008) *Australia's Welfare Wars Revisited*, Sydney: UNSW Press.

Messerschmidt, J. (1993) *Masculinities and Crime*. Lanham, MD: Rowman and Littlefield.

——(1997) *Crime as Structured Action*. Thousand Oaks, CA: Sage.

Michael, Y.L., Berkman, L.F., Colditz, G.A., Holmes, M.D. and Kawachi, I. (2002) 'Social networks and health-related quality of life in breast cancer survivors: a prospective study', *Journal of Psychosomatic Research*, 52: 285–93.

Mickus, M.A. and Luz, C.C. (2002) 'Televisits: sustaining long distance family relationships among institutionalised elders through technology', *Aging and Mental Health*, 6(4): 387–96.

Milbourne, L. (2002) 'Life at the margin: education of young people, social policy and the meanings of social exclusion', *International Journal of Inclusive Education*, 6(4): 325–43.

Miles, M. and Huberman A. (1994) *Qualitative Data Analysis: An Expanded Sourcebook* (2nd edn), Thousand Oaks, CA: Sage.

Millar, J. (2007) 'Social exclusion and social policy research: defining exclusion', in D. Abrams, J. Christian and D. Gordon (eds) *Multidisciplinary Handbook of Social Exclusion Research*, Chichester: John Wiley and Sons.

Miller, J. and Rodwell, M.K. (1997) 'Disclosure of student status in agencies: do we still have a secret?' *Families in Society*, 78: 72–83.

Mills, E.A. (2006) 'From the physical self to the social body: expressions and effects of HIV-related stigma in South Africa', *Journal of Community and Applied Social Psychology*, 16: 498–503.

Minden, S., Frankel, D., Hadden, L., Srinath, K. and Perloff, J. (2004) 'Disability in elderly people with multiple sclerosis: an analysis of baseline data from the Sonya Slifka longitudinal multiple sclerosis study', *NeuroRehabilitation*, 19(1): 55–67.

Minh-ha, T.T. (1988) 'Not you/like you: post-colonial women and the interlocking questions of identity and difference', *Inscriptions*, 3: 71–7.

Ministerial Advisory Committee on Gay and Lesbian Health (2003) *What's The Difference? Health Issues of Major Concern to Gay, Lesbian, Bisexual, Transgender and Intersex (GLBTI) Victorians*, Melbourne: Rural and Regional Health and Aged Care Services Division, Victorian Government Department of Human Services.

Ministry of Social Development (2007) *The Social Report 2007: Indicators of Social Wellbeing in New Zealand*, Wellington: The Ministry of Social Development. Online. Available HTTP: <http://www.socialreport.msd.govt.nz/tools/downloads.html> (accessed 3 January 2009).

Minow, M. (1990) *Making All The Difference: Inclusion, Exclusion and American Law*, New York: Cornell University Press.

Mizielinska, J. (2001) '"The rest is silence … " – Polish nationalism and the question of lesbian existence', *European Journal of Women's Studies*, 8: 281–97.

Moffatt, K. (1999) 'Surveillance and government of the welfare recipient', in A.S. Chambon, A. Irving and L. Epstein (eds) *Reading Foucault for Social Work*, New York: Columbia University Press.

Mohanty, C.T. (1991) 'Under Western eyes: feminist scholarship and colonial discourses', in: C.T. Mohanty, A. Russo and L. Torres (eds) *Third World Women and the Politics of Feminism*, Birmingham: Indiana University Press.

Moore, L.S. and Unwin, C.A. (1991), 'Gatekeeping: a model for screening baccalaureate students for field education', *Journal of Social Work Education*, 27: 8–17.

Morell, C.M. (1994) *Unwomanly Conduct: The Challenges of Intentional Childlessness*, New York: Routledge.

Morgan, C., Burns, T., Fitzpatrick, R., Pinfold, V. and Priebe, S. (2007) 'Social exclusion and mental health', *British Journal of Psychiatry*, 191: 477–83.

Morrow, V. (2001) 'Young people's explanations and experiences of social exclusion: retrieving Bourdieu's concept of social capital', *International Journal of Sociology and Social Policy*, 21(4): 37–63.

Mullaly, B. (2001) 'Confronting the politics of despair: toward the reconstruction of progressive social work in a global economy and postmodern age', *Social Work Education*, 20(3): 303–20.

——(2002) *Challenging Oppression: A Critical Social Work Approach*. Toronto: Oxford University Press.

Mullins, A., McCluskey, J. and Taylor-Browne, J. (2001) *Challenging the Rural Idyll: Children and Families Speak out about Life in Rural England in 21st Century*, London: NCH on behalf of the Countryside Agency.

Narayan, D. and Pritchett, L. (1999) 'Cents and sociability: household income and social capital in rural Tanzania', *Economic Development and Social Change*, 47(4): 871–97.

National Institute on Aging (NIA) and National Institutes of Health (NIH) (2007) *Why Population Aging Matters: A Global Perspective*, Washington, DC: Department of State and the Department of Health and Human Services, National Institute on Aging, National Institutes of Health, Publication No. 07–6134.

Nelson, J.R., Benner, G.J. and Gonzalez, J. (2005) 'An investigation of the effects of a prereading intervention on the early literacy skills of children at risk of emotional disturbance and reading problems', *Journal of Emotional and Behavioural Disorders*, 13: 3–12.

Ng, S.H. (1998) 'Social psychology in an ageing world: ageism and intergenerational relations', *Asian Journal Of Social Psychology*, 1(1): 99–116.

Nicoloupoulou, A. (2005) 'Play and narrative in the process of development: commonalities, differences and interrelations', *Cognitive Development*, 20: 495–502.

Noblit, G. and Hare, R. (1988) *Meta-Ethnography: Synthesizing Qualitative Studies*, Newbury Park, California: Sage Publications.

Notley, T. and Tacchi, J. (2005) 'Online youth networks: researching the experiences of "peripheral" young people in using new media tools for creative participation and representation'. *3C Media Journal of Community, Citizen's and Third Sector Media and Communication*, Issue 1: 73–81. Online E-journal hosted at: <http://www.cbonline.org.au> (accessed 12 April 2007).

NSW Government (2004) *Submission to the Standing Committee on Social Issues-Inquiry into Redfern and Waterloo*, 30 April 2004. Online. Available HTTP: <http://www.redfernwaterloo.nsw.gov.au> (accessed 8 June 2005).

O'Brien, J. (1998) 'Introduction: differences and inequalities', in J. O'Brien and J. Howard (eds) *Everyday Inequalities: Critical Interrogations*, Malden, MA: Blackwell.

Oliver, M. (1996) *Understanding Disability: From Theory to Practice*, Houndsmill: Macmillan Press.

Onyx, J. and Warburton, J. (2003) 'Volunteering and health among older people: a review', *Australasian Journal on Ageing*, 22: 65–9.

O'Reilly, D. (2005) 'Social inclusion: a philosophical anthropology', *Politics*, 25: 80–8.

Organisation for Economic Co-operation and Development (2007) *International Migration Outlook, 2007*, Paris: Sopemi Edition OECD.

Owens, T.J., Stryker, S. and Goodman, N. (2001) *Extending Self-Esteem Theory and Research. Sociological and Psychological Currents*, Cambridge: Cambridge University Press.

Page, E.H. (2004) 'Mental health services experiences of bisexual women and bisexual men: an empirical study', *Journal of Bisexuality*, 4: 137–60.

Page, R. (1984) *Stigma*, London: Routledge and Kegan Paul.

Palermo, G.B. (2001) 'The affective alienation of the elderly – a humane and ethical issue', in D.N. Weisstub, D.C. Thomasma, S. Gauthier and G.F. Tomossy (eds) *Aging: Culture, Health, and Social Change*, Dordrecht: Kluwer Academic Publishers.

Palley, E. (2004) 'Balancing student mental health needs and discipline: implementation of the Individuals with Disabilities Education Act', *Social Service Review*, 78: 243–66.

——(2006) 'Challenges of rights-based law', *Journal of Disability Policy Studies*, 16(4): 229–35.

Pallotta-Chiarolli, M. (2005a) (ed.) *When Our Children Come Out: How to Support Gay, Lesbian, Bisexual and Transgendered Young People*, Sydney: Finch Publishing.

——(2005b) '"We're the X-Files": bisexual students "Messing Up Tidy Sex Files"', in K. Gilbert (ed.) *Sexuality, Sport and the Culture of Risk*, Oxford: Meyer and Meyer.

——(2006) 'On the borders of sexuality research: young people who have sex with both males and females', *Journal of Gay and Lesbian Issues in Education*, 3(2–3): 79–86.

——(2010) *Border Sexualities, Border Families in Schools*, New York: Rowman and Littlefield.

Panagakos, A.N. and Horst, H.A. (2006) 'Return to Cyberia: technology and the social worlds of transnational migrants', *Global Networks*, 6(2): 109–24.

Parish, S. and Huh, J. (2006) 'Health care for women with disabilities: population-based evidence of disparities', *Health and Social Work*, 31(1): 7–15.

Park, K. (2002) 'Stigma management among the voluntary childless', *Sociological Perspectives*, 45: 21–45.

——(2005) 'Choosing childlessness: Weber's typology of action and motives of the voluntary childless', *Sociological Inquiry*, 75: 372–402.

Park, R. and Miller, H. (1921) *Old Word Traits Transplanted*, New York: Arno Press.

Parker, R. and Aggleton, P. (2003) 'HIV and AIDS-related stigma and discrimination: a conceptual framework and implications for action', *Social Science and Medicine*, 57: 13–24.

Parsons, J.T., Kelly, B.C. and Wells, B.C. (2006) 'Differences in club drug use between heterosexual and lesbian/bisexual females', *Addictive Behaviours*, 31: 2344–9.

Patulny, R.V. and Svendsen, G.L.H. (2007) 'Exploring the social capital grid: bonding, bridging, qualitative, quantitative', *International Journal of Sociology and Social Policy*, 27(1): 32–51.

Peace, R. (2001) 'Social exclusion: a concept in need of definition?' *Social Policy Journal of New Zealand*, 16: 17–34.

Pearlin, L., Mullan, J., Semple, S. and Skaff, M. (1990) 'Caregiving and the stress process: an overview of concepts and their measures', *Gerontologist*, 30: 583–94.

Pease, B. (2000) *Recreating Men: Postmodern Masculinity Politics*, London: Sage.

Pellegrini, A.D. and Galda, L. (1993) 'Ten years after: a reexamination of symbolic play and literacy research', *Reading Research Quarterly*, 28: 162–75.

Perez-Escamilla, R. and Putnik, P. (2007) 'The role of acculturation in nutrition, life-style, and incidence of type 2 diabetes among Latinos', *The Journal of Nutrition*, 137: 860–70.

Perry, B. (2001) *In the Name of Hate: Understanding Hate Crimes*, New York: Routledge.

Perry, R.W. (2004), 'The impact of criminal conviction disclosure on the self-reported offending profile of social work students', *British Journal of Social Work*, 34: 997–1008.

Peterson, A.R. (1994) *In a Critical Condition: Health and Power Relations in Australia*, St Leonards, NSW: Allen and Unwin.

Petros, G., Airhihenbuwa, C., Simbayi, L. Ramlagan, S. and Brown, B. (2006) 'HIV/AIDS and "othering" in South Africa: the blame goes on', *Culture, Health and Sexuality*, 8(1): 67–77.

Pfeffer, N. (2004) 'Screening for breast cancer: candidacy and compliance', *Social Science and Medicine*, 58: 151–60.

Pheterson, G. (1986) 'Alliances between women: overcoming internalised oppression and internalised domination', *Signs: Journal of Women in Culture and Society*, 12 (1): 146–60.

Piachaud, D. (2002) *Capital and the Determinants of Poverty and Social Exclusion*, London: CASE Papers 60, Centre for Analysis of Social Exclusion, LSE.

Pickering, M. (2001) *Stereotyping: The Politics of Representation*, Basingstoke: Palgrave.

Pierson, J. (2001) *Tackling Social Exclusion*, London: Routledge.

Pinker, R. (1989), 'Social work and social policy in the twentieth century: retrospect and prospect', in M. Bulmer, J. Lewis and D. Piachaud (eds) *The Goals of Social Policy*, London: Unwin Hyman.

Pluss, M. (2004) 'Digital divide in Australia', *Geography Bulletin*, 36(4): 56–9.

Pollock, S. (2008) *Background Paper for Wesley Mission Melbourne Social Inclusion Policy*, Melbourne: Wesley Mission Melbourne.

Poole, M. (2000) 'Socialisation', in R. Jureidini and M. Poole (eds) *Sociology: Australian Connections*, St Leonards: Allen and Unwin.

Popay, J., Escorel, S., Hernández, M., Johnston, H., Mathieson, J. and Rispel, L. (2008) *Understanding and Tackling Social Exclusion. Final Report to the WHO Commission on Social Determinants of Health from the Social Exclusion Knowledge Network*, February 2008. Online. Available HTTP: <http://www.who.int/social_determinants/knowledge_networks/final_reports/sekn_final%20report_042008.pdf> (accessed 27 June 2008).

Portes, A. (1998) 'Social capital: its origins and applications in modern sociology', *Annual Review of Sociology*, 98(24): 1–24.

Portnoy, K.E. and Berry, J.M. (1997) 'Mobilizing minority communities: social capital and participation in urban neighbourhoods', *American Behavioral Scientist*, 40(5): 632–44.

Power, A. and Wilson, W.J. (2000) *Social Exclusion and the Future of Cities*, London: Centre for the Analysis of Social Exclusion Paper 35. Online. Available HTTP: <http://sticerd.lse.ac.uk/dps/case/cp/CASEpaper35.pdf> (accessed 16 November 2007).

Pressey, N.K. and Holm, S.M. (2006) *Building Successful Schools and Leaders in High Poverty Communities*, Online. Available HTTP: <http://209.85.165.104/search?q=cache:vgZL-4cZ5h8J:www.wm.edu/education/599/0> (accessed 25 February 2008).

Prislin, R., Suarez, L., Simpson, D.M. and Dyer, J (1998) 'When acculturation hurts: the case of immunization', *Social Science and Medicine* 47: 1947–56.

Probyn, Elspeth (1996) *Outside Belongings*, New York: Routledge.

Puri, S.K. and Sahay, S. (2003) 'Participation through communicative action: a case study of GIS for addressing land/water development in India', *Information Technology for Development*, 10: 179–99.

Putnam, M., Greenen, S., Powers, L., Saxton, M., Finney, S. and Dautel, P. (2003) 'Health and wellness: people with disabilities discuss barriers and facilitators to well being', *Journal of Rehabilitation*, 69(1): 37–45.

Putnam, R.D. (1993) *Making Democracy Work: Civic Traditions in Modern Italy*, Princeton NJ: Princeton University Press.

——(2000) *Bowling Alone: The Collapse and Revival of American Community*, New York: Simon and Schuster.

Raco, M. (2002) 'The social relations of organisational activity and the new local governance in the UK', *Urban Studies*, 39(3): 437–56.

Randolph, B. and Judd, B. (2000) 'Community renewal and large public housing estates', *Urban Policy and Research*, 18(1): 91–104.

Randolph, B. and Holloway, D. (2004) *Social Disadvantage, Tenure and Location: An Analysis of Sydney and Melbourne*, Research Paper No.12, NSW: University of Western Sydney, Urban Frontiers Program.

Rawls, J. (1971) *A Theory of Justice*, Cambridge, MA: Harvard University Press.

Razack, S. (1998) *Looking White People in the Eye*, Toronto: University of Toronto Press.

Reed, D., McGee, D., Cohen, J., Yano, K., Syme, S and Feinleib, M. (1982) 'Acculturation and coronary heart disease among Japanese men in Hawaii', *American Journal of Epidemiology*, 115: 894–905.

Reid, C. (2004) *The Wounds of Exclusion: Poverty, Women's Health and Social Justice*, Edmonton: International Institute for Qualitative Methodology Press.

Reid, W. and Caswell, D. (2005) 'A national telephone and online counselling service for young Australians', in R. Wootton and J. Batch (eds) *Telepediatrics: Telemedicine and Child Health*, London: The Royal Society of Medicine Press Ltd.

Reidpath, D.D., Chan, K.Y., Gifford, S.M. and Allotey, P. (2005) 'He hath the French pox: stigma, social value and social exclusion', *Sociology of Health and Illness*, 27: 468–89.

Renner, S., Prewitt, G., Watanabe, M. and Gascho, L. (2007) *Summary of the Virtual Round Table on Social Exclusion*, Poverty, HDR and Crisis Prevention and Recovery Networks. Online. Available HTTP: <http://hdr.undp.org/en/nhdr/knowledgenetworks/replies/161.pdf > (accessed 24 October 2007).

Renzaho, A.M.N. (2002) *Addressing the Needs of Refugees and Humanitarian Entrants in Victoria: An Evaluation of Health and Community Services*, Richmond, Victoria: Centre for Culture Ethnicity and Health.

Renzaho, A. (2007) 'Providing health services to migrants and refugees settling in Victoria, Australia: an analysis of the complexity, cost and policy implications for public health', *International Journal of Migration, Health and Social Care*, 3(4): 31–43.

——(2008) 'Re-visioning cultural competence in community health services in Victoria', *Australian Health Review*, 32(2): 223–35.

Rich, A. (1987) *Blood, Bread and Poetry*, London: Virago.

Richardson, L. and Le Grand, J. (2002) *Outsider and Insider Expertise: The Response of Residents of Deprived Neighbourhoods to an Academic Definition of Social Exclusion*, CASE, LSE, London: Centre for the Analysis of Social Exclusion Paper 57. Online. Available HTTP: <http://sticerd.lse.ac.uk/dps/case/cp/CASEpaper35.pdf> (accessed 25 November 2007).

Richter, L.M., van Rooyen, H., Solomon, V., Griesel, D. and Durrheim, K. (2001) 'Putting HIV/AIDS counselling in South Africa in its place', *Society in Transition*, 32(1): 148–54

Ring, I.T. and Wenitong, M. (2007) 'Interventions to halt child abuse in Aboriginal communities', *Medical Journal of Australia*, 187: 204–5.

Roach, S., Atkinson, D., Waters, A. and Jefferies, F. (2007) 'Primary health care in the Kimberley: is the doctor shortage much bigger than we think?', *Australian Journal of Rural Health*, 15(6): 373–9.

Robin, L., Brener, N.D., Donahue, S.F., Hack, T., Hale, K. and Goodenow, C. (2002) 'Association between health risk behaviors and opposite-, same-, and both-sex sexual partners in representative samples of Vermont and Massachusetts high school students', *Archives of Pediatrics and Adolescent Medicine*, 156: 349–56.

Rokach, A., Matalon, R., Rokach, B. and Safarov, A. (2007) 'The effects of gender and marital status on loneliness of the aged', *Social Behavior and Personality*, 35(2): 243–54.

Rönneling, A. and Gabàs i Gasa, À. (2007) 'Welfare or what? Conditions for coping within different socio-political structures: the examples of Sweden and Spain', in H. Steinert and A. Pilgram (eds) *Welfare Policy from Below: Struggles Against Social Exclusion in Europe*, Aldershot: Ashgate.

Room, G. (1995) 'Poverty and social exclusion: the new European agenda for policy research', in G. Room (ed.) *Beyond the Threshold, The Measurement and Analysis of Social Exclusion*, Bristol: Bristol Policy Press.

——(1999) 'Social exclusion, solidarity and the challenge of globalization', *International Journal of Social Welfare*, 8(3): 166–74.

Room, G.J. and Britton, N. (2006) 'The dynamics of social exclusion', *International Journal of Social Welfare*, 15(4): 280–9.

Rorty, R. (1989) *Contingency, Irony and Solidarity*, Cambridge: Cambridge University Press

Rosario, M., Schrimshaw, E.W. and Hunter, J. (2004) 'Predictors of substance use over time among gay, lesbian and bisexual youths: an examination of three hypotheses', *Addictive Behaviours*, 29: 1623–31.

Rosenberg, M. (1979) *Conceiving of the Self*, New York: Basic Books.

Rosenblum, K.E. and Travis, T. (1996) 'Experiencing difference: framework essay', in K.E. Rosenblum (ed.) *The Meaning of Difference: American Constructions of Race, Sex and Gender, Social Class and Sexual Orientation*, New York: McGraw-Hill.

Rosenfeld, E.R. (1997) *Social Support and Health Status: A Literature Review*, Adelaide: South Australian Community Health Research Unit.

Roth, D.L., Mittleman, M.S., Clay, O.J., Madan, A. and Haley, W.E. (2005) 'Changes in social support as mediators of the impact of a psychosocial intervention for spouse caregivers of persons with Alzheimer's disease', *Psychology and Aging*, 20: 634–44.

Rudmin, W. (2006) 'Debate in science: the case of acculturation', *AnthroGlobe Journal*. Online. Available HTTP: <http://malinowski.kent.ac.uk/docs/rudminf_acculturation_061204.pdf > (accessed 20 January 2008).

Russell, A. and Perris, K. (2003) 'Telementoring in community nursing: a shift from dyadic to communal models of learning and professional development', *Mentoring and Tutoring*, 11(2): 227–37.

Russell, B. (1951) *Unpopular Essays*, London: Allen and Unwin.

Russell, P. (2003) 'Access and achievement or social exclusion? Are the government's policies working for disabled children and their families?', *Children and Society*, 17 (3): 215–25.

Russell, S.T. and Seif, H. (2002) 'Bisexual female adolescents: a critical analysis of past research and results from a national survey', *Journal of Bisexuality*, 2(2/3): 73–94.

Russo, F.N. (1979) 'Overview: sex roles, fertility and the motherhood mandate', *Psychology of Women Quarterly*, 41: 7–12.

Ryan, K. (2007) *Social Exclusion and the Politics of Order*, Manchester: Manchester University Press.

Sacks, V. (1996) 'Women and AIDS: an analysis of media misrepresentations', *Social Science and Medicine*, 42: 59–73.

Sampson, R.J. (1991) 'Linking the micro- and macrolevel dimensions of community social organization', *Social Forces*, 70(1): 43–64.

Sanchez-Jankowski, M. (1999) 'The concentration of African-American poverty and the dispersal of the working class', *International Journal of Urban and Regional Research*, 23: 619–37.

Saraceno, C. (2001) 'Social exclusion, cultural roots and diversities of a popular concept', Conference on Social Exclusion and Children, Institute for Child and Family Policy. Online. Available HTTP: <http://www.childpolicyintl.org/publications/Saraceno.pdf> (accessed 1 August 2007).

Saunders, P., Naidoo, Y. and Griffiths, M. (2007) *Towards New Indicators of Disadvantage: Deprivation and Social Exclusion in Australia*, Sydney: Social Policy Research Centre.

Savin-Williams, R. (2005) *The New Gay Teenager*, Cambridge, MA: Harvard University Press.

Sawhney, S. (1995) 'The joke and the hoax: (not) speaking as the Other', in J. Roof and R. Wiegman (eds) *Who Can Speak? Authority and Critical Identity*. Chicago: University of Illinois Press.

Schacht, R. (1971) *Alienation*, New York: Doubleday and Company Inc.

Schaefer, K. (2006) 'Market-based solutions for improving telecommunications access and choice for consumers with disabilities', *Journal of Disability Policy Studies*, 17(2): 116–26.

Scheer, J., Kroll, T., Neri, M. and Beatty, P. (2003) 'Access barriers for persons with disabilities: the consumer's perspective', *Journal of Disability Policy Studies*, 13(4): 221–30.

Schofield, H., Bloch, S., Herrman, H., Murphy, B., Nankervis, J. and Singh, B. (1998) *Family Caregivers: Disability, Illness and Ageing*, St Leonards, NSW: Allen and Unwin.

Schreiber R., Crooks D. and Stern P. (1997) 'Qualitative meta-analysis', in J. Morse (ed.) *Completing a Qualitative Project: Details and Dialogue*, Thousand Oaks, CA: Sage.

Schuller, T., Baron, S. and Field, J. (2000) 'Social capital, a review and a critique', in S. Baron, J. Field and T. Schuller (eds) *Social Capital: Critical Perspectives*, Oxford: Oxford University Press.

Schutte, G. (2000) 'Being African in South Africa: the dynamics of exclusion and inclusion', *Social Identities*, 6(2): 207–22.

Schwalbe, M., Godwin, S., Holden, D., Schrock, D., Thompson, S. and Wolkomir, M. (2000) 'Generic processes in the reproduction of inequality: an interactionist approach', *Social Forces*, 79: 419–52.

Schweinhart, L., Barnes, H., Weikart, D. and Barnett, W. (1993) *Significant Benefits: The High/Scope Perry Preschool Study Through Age 27*, Michigan: High/Scope Press.

Scott, N. and Zeiger, S. (2000) 'Should convicted felons be denied admission to a social work education program? No!' *Journal of Social Work Education*, 36: 409–11.

Scott, S. (1999) 'Fragmented selves in late modernity: making sociological sense of multiple personalities', *The Sociological Review*, 47: 432–60.

Seccombe, K. (1991) 'Assessing the costs and benefits of children: gender comparisons among childfree husbands and wives', *Journal of Marriage and the Family*, 53: 191–202.

Seeman, M. (1959) 'On the meaning of alienation', *American Sociological Review*, 24(6): 783–91.

Selwyn, N. (2002) '"E-stablishing" an inclusive society? Technology, social exclusion and UK government policy making', *Journal of Social Policy*, 31(1): 1–20.

Sen, A. (2000) 'Social exclusion: concept, application, and scrutiny', Social Development Paper No 1, Office of Environment and Social Development Asian Development Bank. Online, Available HTTP: <http://www.adb.org/documents/books/social_exclusion/Social_exclusion.pdf> (accessed 1 August 2007).

Shah, M., Zhu, K. and Potter, J. (2006) 'Hispanic acculturation and utilization of colorectal cancer screening in the United States', *Cancer Detection and Prevention*, 30: 306–12.

Shardlow, S. (2000) 'Legal responsibility and liability in fieldwork', in L. Cooper and L. Briggs (eds) *Fieldwork in the Human Services*, St Leonards: Allen and Unwin.

Sheldon, T.A. (2005) 'Making evidence synthesis more useful for management and policy-making', *Journal of Health Services Research and Policy*, 10 (supp. 1): 1–5.

Sheldrake, P. (2001) 'Human identity and the particularity of place', *Spiritus*, 1(1): 43–64.

Sheppard, M. (2006) *Social Work and Social Exclusion: The Idea of Practice*, Aldershot: Ashgate.

Sidanius, J. and Pratto, F. (1999) *Social Dominance: An Intergroup Theory of Social Hierarchy and Oppression*, Cambridge: Cambridge University Press.

Silveira, E. and Allebeck, P. (2001) 'Migration, ageing and mental health: an ethnographic study on perceptions of life satisfaction, anxiety and depression in older Somali men in east London', *International Journal of Social Welfare*, 10: 309–20.

Silver, H. (1994) 'Social exclusion and social solidarity: three paradigms', *International Labour Review*, 133(5–6): 531–48.

Silverman, D. (2001) *Interpreting Qualitative Data: Methods for Analysing Talk, Text and Interaction* (2nd edn), London: Sage.

Simmonds, G. (2000) 'Traditions of spiritual guidance: spiritual direction in cyberspace', *The Way*, 40(3): 263–71.

Singer, L. (1993) *Erotic Welfare: Sexual Theory and Politics in the Age of Epidemic*, New York, London: Routledge.

Singh, J.A., Govender, M. and Mills, E. J. (2007) 'Do human rights matter to health?' *The Lancet*, 370: 521–7.

Skinner, D. and Mfecane, S. (2004) 'Stigma, discrimination and the implications for people living with HIV/AIDS in South Africa', *Journal of Social Aspects of HIV/ AIDS*, 1(3): 157–64.

Sloop, J.M. (2005) 'In a queer time and place and race: instersectionality comes of age', *Quarterly Journal of Speech* 91(3): 312–26.

Smart, M. (2004) 'Transition planning and the needs of young people and their carers: the alumni project', *British Journal of Special Education*, 31(3): 128–37.

Smedley, B.D. and Syme, S.L. (2001) *Promoting Health Intervention Strategies from Social and Behavioral Research*, Washington DC: National Academy Press.

Smith, D. and Stewart, D. (1998) 'Probation and social exclusion', in C. Jones Finer and M. Nellis (eds) *Crime and Social Exclusion*, Oxford: Blackwell Publishers.

Smith, E., Murray, S., Yousafzai, A. and Kasonka, L. (2004) 'Barriers to accessing safe motherhood and reproductive health services: the situation of women with disabilities in Lusaka, Zambia', *Disability and Rehabilitation*, 26(2): 121–7.

Smith, J.M. (1999), 'Prior criminality and employment of social workers with substantial access to children: a decision board analysis', *British Journal of Social Work*, 29: 49–68.

Smith, J., Brooks-Gunn, J., Klebanov, P. and Lee, K. (2000) 'Welfare and work: complementary strategies for low-income women?' *Journal of Marriage and Family*, 62: 808–21.

Smith, S.J., Easterlow, D., Munro, M. and Turner, K.M. (2003) 'Housing as health capital: how health trajectories and housing paths are linked', *Journal of Social Issues*, 59(3): 501–25.

Snow, C.E., Scarborough, H.S. and Burns, M.S. (1999) 'What speech-language pathologists need to know about early reading', *Topics in Language Disorders*, 20: 48–58.

Social Exclusion Unit and Cabinet Office (2001) *What is Social Exclusion?* London: Cabinet Office.

Solis, J., Marks, G., Garcia, M. and Shelton, D. (1990) 'Acculturation, access to care, and use of preventive services by Hispanics: findings from Hanes 1982–84', *American Journal of Public Health*, 80: 1–19.

Somerville, P. (1998) 'Explanations of social exclusion: where does housing fit in?' *Housing Studies*, 13(6): 761–80.

——(2000) *Social Relations and Social Exclusion*, London: Routledge.

Song, L., Biegel, D. and Milligan, S. (1997) 'Predictors of depressive symptomology among lower social class caregivers of persons with chronic mental illness', *Community Mental Health Journal*, 33: 269–86.

Sooman, A. and Macintyre, S. (1995) 'Health and perceptions of the local environment in socially contrasting neighborhoods in Glasgow', *Health and Place*, 1(1): 15–26.

Spandler, H. (2007) 'From social exclusion to inclusion? A critique of the inclusion imperative in mental health', *Medical Sociology Online*, 2(2): 3–16.

Squire, C. (2007) *HIV in South Africa: Talking about the Big Thing*, London: Routledge.

Srinivasan, R. (2006) 'Where information society and community voice intersect', *The Information Society*, 22: 355–65.

Stafford, M., Bartley, M., Sacker, A., Marmot, M., Wilkinson, R., Boreham, R. and Thomas, R. (2003) 'Measuring the social environment: social cohesion and material deprivation in English and Scottish neighbourhoods', *Environment and Planning A*, 35: 1459–75.

Stagnitti, K. and Jennings, C. (2007) *The Effectiveness of the Reading Discovery Program as an Intervention to Increase Literacy and Social Inclusion for Marginalised Children: A Pilot Study*, Geelong, Victoria: Deakin University, School of Health and Social Development, Occupational Science and Therapy.

State Government of Victoria, Department of Human Services (2007) 'Dental health services Victoria – information and communications technology project'. Online. Available HTTP: <http://www.health.vic.gov.au/healthsmart/dhsv.htm> (accessed 25 February 2008).

Stavenhagen, R. (2005) 'The situation of human rights and fundamental freedoms of indigenous people', Commission on Human Rights E/CN.4/2005/88. Online. Available HTTP: <http://daccessdds.un.org/doc/UNDOC/GEN/G05/101/57/PDF/G0510157.pdf?OpenElement> (accessed 1 December 2008).

Steinert, H. (2007a) 'The cultures of welfare and exclusion', in H. Steinert and A. Pilgram (eds) *Welfare Policy from Below: Struggles Against Social Exclusion in Europe*, Aldershot: Ashgate.

Steinert, H. (2007b) 'Participation and social exclusion: a conceptual framework', in H. Steinert and A. Pilgram (eds) *Welfare Policy from Below: Struggles Against Social Exclusion in Europe*, Aldershot: Ashgate.

Steinert H. and Pilgram A. (eds) (2007) *Welfare Policy from Below: Struggles Against Social Exclusion in Europe*, Aldershot: Ashgate.

Stein-Roggenbuck, S. (2005), '"Wholly within the discretion of the probate court": judicial authority and Mother's Pensions in Michigan, 1913–40', *Social Service Review*, 79: 294–321.

Strauss, A. and Corbin, J. (1998) *Basics of Qualitative Research: Techniques and Procedures for Developing Grounded Theory* (2nd edn), Thousand Oaks: Sage.

Sullivan, H. (2002) 'Modernization, neighbourhood management and social inclusion', *Public Management Review*, 4(4): 505–28.

Sung, K-T. and Kim, H.S. (2003) 'Elder respect among young adults: exploration of behavioral forms in Korea', *Ageing International*, 28(3): 279–94.

Szreter, S. and Woolcock, M. (2004) 'Health by association? Social capital, social theory and the political economy of public health', *International Journal of Epidemiology*, 33: 650–67.

Tajfel, H. and Turner, J.C. (1986) 'The social identity theory of intergroup behaviour', in S. Worshel and W. Austin (eds) *Psychology of Intergroup Relations*, Nelson Hall: Chicago.

Takács, J. (2006) 'Social exclusion of young lesbian, gay, bisexual and transgender (LGBT) people in Europe', Brussels: ILGA-Europe and IGLYO. Online. Available HTTP: <http://www.equalisnotenough.org/followup/papers/Paradis%20&%20Takacs,%20Report%20-%20Social%20exclusion%20of%20young%20LGBT%20people.pdf> (accessed 10 October 2008).

Taket, A. (2001) *Health-related Services for Women: The Views of Somali Women Living in Redbridge and Waltham Forest*, London: London South Bank University.

Taket, A. and Barter-Godfrey, S. (2005) *Women and Health: Views of Women aged 50–64, living in Lambeth, Southwark and Lewisham (with a Focus on Breast Cancer Screening)*, London: Institute of Primary Care and Public Health, London South Bank University.

——(2007) 'Understanding women's breast screening behaviour: a study carried out in South East London with women aged 50–64 years', *Health Education Journal*, 66: 335–46.

Taket, A.R., Beringer, A., Irvine, A. and Garfield, S. (2004) *Tackling Domestic Violence: Exploring the Health Service Contribution. Evaluation of the Crime Reduction Programme Violence Against Women Initiative Health Projects*, Home Office Online Report 52/04. Online. Available HTTP: <http://www.homeoffice.gov.uk/rds/pdfs04/rdsolr5204.pdf> (accessed 31 July 2008).

Tamm, M. and Prellwitz, M. (2001) 'If I had a friend in a wheelchair: children's thoughts on disabilities', *Child: Care, Health and Development*, 27(3): 223–40.

Tang, K-L. and Lee, J-J. (2006) 'Global social justice for older people: the case for an international convention on the rights of older people', *British Journal of Social Work*, 36(7): 1135–50.

Taylor, R. and Lee, H. (2005) 'Occupational therapists perception of usage of information and communication technology (ICT) in Western Australia and the association of availability of ICT on recruitment and retention of therapists working in rural areas', *Australian Occupation Therapy Journal*, 52: 51–6.

Taxman, F.S., Young, D. and Byrne, J.M. (2002) *Offender's Views of Reentry: Implications for Processes, Programs and Services*, College Park: University of Maryland, Bureau of Governmental Research. Online. Available HTTP: <http://bgr.umn.edu> (accessed 27 June 2006).

Teychenne, M., Ball, K. and Salmon, J. (2008) 'Physical activity and likelihood of depression in adults: a review', *Preventive Medicine*, 46: 397–411.

Thomas, C. (2004) 'How is disability understood? An examination of sociological approaches', *Disability and Society*, 19(6): 569–83.

Thomas, P. (2004) 'The experience of disabled people as customers in the owner occupation market', *Housing Studies*, 19(5): 781–94.

Thorne, B. (2002) 'Symposium on West and Fenstermaker's "Doing Difference"', in S. Fenstermaker and C. West (eds) *Doing Difference, Doing Gender: Inequality, Power and Institutional Change*, New York: Routledge.

Thorpe, D. (1994) *Evaluating Child Protection*, Buckingham: Open University Press.

Tillner, G. (1997) 'Masculinity and xenophobia: the identity of dominance', paper presented to the UNESCO conference, *Masculinity and Male Roles in the Perspective of a Culture of Peace*, Oslo, Norway.

Tippin, D. and Baker, M. (2002) 'Managing the health of the poor: contradictions in welfare-to-work programs', *Just Policy*, 28: 33–41.

Tjaden, P. and Thoennes, N. (2000) *Extent, Nature, and Consequences of Intimate Partner Violence: Findings from the National Violence Against Women Survey*. Washington: US Dept of Justice.

Todman, L. (2004) *Reflections on Social Exclusion: What is it? How is it Different from US Conceptualizations of Disadvantage? And, Why Might Americans Consider Integrating it into US Social Policy Discourse?* City Futures: an international conference on globalism and urban change, Chicago, US, 8–10 July 2004. Online. Available HTTP: <http://www.uic.edu/cuppa/cityfutures/papers/webpapers/cityfuturespapers/session2_3/2_3reflections.pdf> (accessed 1 July 2008).

Torres, S. (2003) 'A preliminary empirical test of a culturally-relevant theoretical framework for the study of successful aging', *Journal of Cross-Cultural Gerontology*, 18: 79–100.

Townsend, S. (2006) *Queen Camilla*, Camberwell: Michael Joseph.

Train, B., Dalton, P. and Elkin, J. (2000) 'Embracing inclusion: the critical role of the library', *Library Management*, 21(9): 483–90.

Travers, M.A. and O'Brien, C. (1997) 'The complexities of bisexual youth identities', in M. Schneider (ed.) *Pride and Prejudice: Working with Lesbian, Gay and Bisexual Youth*, Toronto: Central Toronto Youth Services.

Triandafyllidou, A. (2003) 'Immigration policy implementation in Italy: organisational culture, identity processes and labour market control', *Journal of Ethnic and Migration Studies*, 29: 257–97.

Tsugane, S. (2005) 'Salt, salted food intake, and risk of gastric cancer: epidemiological evidence', *Cancer Science*, 96: 1–6.

Twigg, J. and Atkin, K. (1994) *Carers Perceived: Policy and Practice in Informal Care*, Buckingham: Open University Press.

Udry, J.R. and Chantala, K. (2002) 'Risk assessment of adolescents with same-sex relationships', *Journal of Adolescent Health*, 31: 84–92.

Ulvestad, A. (2006) 'The health and well-being of older women in rural Victoria: an evaluation of the relationship between social connectedness and mental health in older adults', Unpublished Bachelor of Occupational Therapy Honours thesis, Deakin University, Australia.

Van Der Geest, S. (1994)'"They don't come to listen": The experience of loneliness among older people in Kwahu, Ghana', *Journal of Cross-Cultural Gerontology*, 19: 77–96.

Van der Westhuizen, J. (2008) 'Popular culture, discourse and divergent identities: reconstructing South Africa as an African state', *African Identities*, 6(1): 45–61.

Van Winden, W. (2001) 'The end of social exclusion? On information technology policy as a key to social inclusion in large European cities', *Regional Studies*, 35(9): 861–8.

Veevers, J.E. (1974) 'Voluntary childlessness and social policy: an alternative view', *The Family Coordinator*, 23: 397–406.

VicHealth (2005) *Social Inclusion as a Determinant of Mental Health and Wellbeing*, Research Summary 2. Melbourne: Mental Health and Wellbeing Unit.

Viet-Wilson, J. (1998) *Setting Adequacy Standards*, Bristol: Policy Press.

Villa, R., Van Tac, L., Muc, P., Ryan, S., Thuy, N., Weill, C. and Thousand, J. (2003) 'Inclusion in Viet Nam: more than a decade of implementation', *Research and Practice for Persons with Severe Disabilities*, 28(1): 23.

von Faber, M., Bootsma-van der Wiehl, A., van Exel, E., Gusselkloo, J., Lagaay, A. M., van Dongen, E., Knook, D., van der Geest, S. and Westendorp, R. (2001) 'Successful aging in the oldest old: who can be characterized as successfully aged?', *Archives of Internal Medicine*, 161: 2694–2700.

Vygotsky, L.S. (1997) *Thought and Language*, Translation Alex Kozulin, Massachusetts: MIT Press.

Waldfogel, J. (1994) 'The effect of criminal conviction on income and the trust "reposed in workmen"', *Journal of Human Resources*, 29: 62–81.

Walker, A. and Walker, C. (eds) (1997) *Britain Divided: The Growth of Social Exclusion in the 1980s and 1990s*, London: Child Poverty Action Group.

Wallerstein, N. (2006) *What is the Evidence on Effectiveness of Empowerment to Improve Health?* Copenhagen: WHO Regional Office for Europe (Health Evidence Network report). Online. Available HTTP: <http://www.euro.who.int/Document/E88086.pdf> (accessed 5 December 2006).

Walter, M. (2002) 'Working their way out of poverty? Sole motherhood, welfare and material well-being', *Journal of Sociology*, 38: 361–80.

Warner, J., McKeown, E., Griffin, M., Johnson, K., Ramsay, A., Cort, C. and King, M. (2004) 'Rates and predictors of mental health in gay men, lesbians, and bisexual men and women: results from a survey based in England and Wales', *British Journal of Psychiatry*, 185: 479–85.

Wassenberg, F. (2004) 'Editorial "Large social housing estates: from stigma to demolition?"' *Journal of Housing and the Built Environment*, 19: 223–32.

Waters, A. (2001) *Do Housing Conditions Impact on Health Inequalities Between Australia's Rich and Poor?* Canberra: Australian Housing and Urban Research Institute-Australian National University Research Centre.

Watt, P. and Jacobs, K. (2000) 'Discourses of social exclusion. an analysis of bringing Britain together: a national strategy for neighbourhood renewal', *Housing, Theory and Society*, 17: 14–26.

Way, J. and Webb, C. (2007) 'A framework for analysing ICT adoption in Australian Primary Schools', *Australian Journal of Educational Technology*, 23(4): 559–82.

Weber, L. (2002) 'Symposium on West and Fenstermaker's "Doing Difference"', in S. Fenstermaker and C. West (eds) *Doing Difference, Doing Gender: Inequality, Power and Institutional Change*, New York: Routledge.

Weeks, J. (1995) 'History, desire, identities', in R.G. Parker and J.H. Gagnon (eds) *Conceiving Sexuality: Approaches to Sex Research in a Postmodern World*, New York: Routledge.

Weis, L. (1995) 'Identity formation and the process of "othering": unravelling sexual threads', *Educational Foundations*, 9: 17–33.

Weiss, D. (ed.) (2003) *Social Exclusion: An Approach To The Australian Case*, New York: Peter Lang Pub Inc.

Wells, C.G. (1985a) *Language Development in the Pre-School Years*, Cambridge: Cambridge University Press.

——(1985b) 'Preschool literacy related activities and later success in school', in D.R. Olson, N. Torrence and A. Hildyard (eds) *Literacy, Language and Learning: The Nature and Consequences of Reading and Writing*, Cambridge: Cambridge University Press.

——(1987) *The Meaning Makers*, London: Hodder and Stoughton.

Wells, L.E. (2001) 'Self-esteem and social inequality' in T.J. Owens, S. Stryker and N. Goodman (eds) *Extending Self-Esteem Theory and Research*, Cambridge: Cambridge University Press.

Welshman, J. (2006a) 'From the cycle of deprivation to social exclusion: five countries', *The Political Quarterly*, 77(4): 475–84.

——(2006b) 'Searching for social capital: historical perspectives on health, poverty and culture', *The Journal of the Royal Society for the Promotion of Health*, 126(6): 268–74.

Wen, M., Cagney, K. and Christakis, N. (2005) 'Effect of specific aspects of community social environment on the mortality of individuals diagnosed with serious illness', *Social Science and Medicine*, 61: 1119–34.

Whinnett, E. (2005) 'High-rise harmony is making sense', *The Herald Sun*, 20/05/2005, p.15.

Wildman, S. and Davis, A. (2000) 'Language and silence: makings systems of privilege visible', in R. Delgado and J. Stefancic (eds) *Critical Race Theory: The Cutting Edge*, 2nd edn, Philadelphia: Temple University Press.

Williams, G. (2001) 'Theorizing disability', in G. Albrecht, K. Seelman and M. Bury (eds) *Handbook of Disability Studies*, Thousand Oaks: Sage.

Williams, J. (2005) 'Designing neighbourhoods for social interaction: the case of cohousing', *Journal of Urban Design*, 10(2): 195–277.

Williams, K.D., Von Hippel, W. and Forgas, J.P. (eds) (2005) *The Social Outcast: Ostracism, Social Exclusion, Rejection, and Bullying*, New York: Psychology Press Ltd.

Williamson, D.L. and Salkie, F. (2005) 'Welfare reforms in Canada: implications for the well-being of pre-school children in poverty', *Journal of Children in Poverty*, 11: 55–76.

Wilson, L. (2004) 'Towards equality: the voices of young disabled people in Disability Rights Commission research', *Support for Learning*, 19(4): 162–8.

Wilson, L. (2006) 'Developing a model for the measurement of social inclusion and social capital in regional Australia', *Social Indicators Research*, 75: 335–60.

Wilson, R. (1997) *Bringing Them Home: Report of the National Inquiry into the Separation of Aboriginal and Torres Strait Islander Children from their Families*, Sydney: Human Rights and Equal Opportunity Commission.

Wilson, W.J. (1987) *The Truly Disadvantaged*, Chicago: University of Chicago Press.

Wonders, N. (2000) 'Conceptualising difference', in the Criminal Justice Collective of Northern Arizona University (eds) *Investigating Difference: Human and Cultural Relations in Criminal Justice*, Boston: Allyn and Bacon.

Wood, L., Giles-Corti, B. and Bulsara, M. (2005) 'The pet connection: pets as a conduit for social capital?' *Social Science and Medicine*, 61: 1159–73.

Woolcock, M. (1998) 'Social capital and economic development: towards a theoretical synthesis and policy framework', *Theory and Society*, 27: 151–208.

World Health Organization (WHO) (2002) 'Towards a common language for functioning, disability and health', Geneva: World Health Organization.

Wynhausen, E. (2008) 'Welcome to work around the clock', *The Weekend Australian, Inquirer*, February 16–17 2008, 26.

Yang, L.H., Kleinman, A., Link, B.G., Phelan, J., Lee, S. and Good, B. (2007) 'Culture and stigma: adding moral experience to stigma theory', *Social Science and Medicine*, 24: 1524–35.

Yeh, S.C. and Lo, S.K. (2004) 'Living alone, social support, and feeling lonely among the elderly', *Social Behavior and Personality*, 32(2): 129–38.

Yewah, E. (2008) 'Undoing and reconstructing African identities: a cultural approach', *African Identities*, 6(1): 17–28.

Young, I.M. (1990) *Justice and the Politics of Difference*, Princeton: Princeton University Press.

Young, J. (n.d.) *Social Exclusion*. Online. Available HTTP: <http://www.malcolmread.co.uk/JockYoung/social_exclusion.pdf > (accessed 20 December 2007).

Young, J. (1998) 'From inclusive to exclusive society: nightmares in the European dream', in V. Ruggerio, N. South and I. Taylor (eds) *The New European Criminology: Crime and Social Order in Europe*, London: Routledge.

Yun, R.J. and Lachman, M.E. (2006) 'Perceptions of aging in two cultures: Korean and American views on old age', *Journal of Cross-Cultural Gerontology*, 21: 55–70.

Zungu-Dirwayi, N., Shinsana, O., Louw, J. and Dana, P. (2007) 'Social determinants for HIV prevalence among South African educators', *AIDS Care*, 19(10): 1296–303.

Index

CPSIA information can be obtained
at www.ICGtesting.com
Printed in the USA
FFOW01n2143030116
19862FF